2010

The Mirror of Yoga

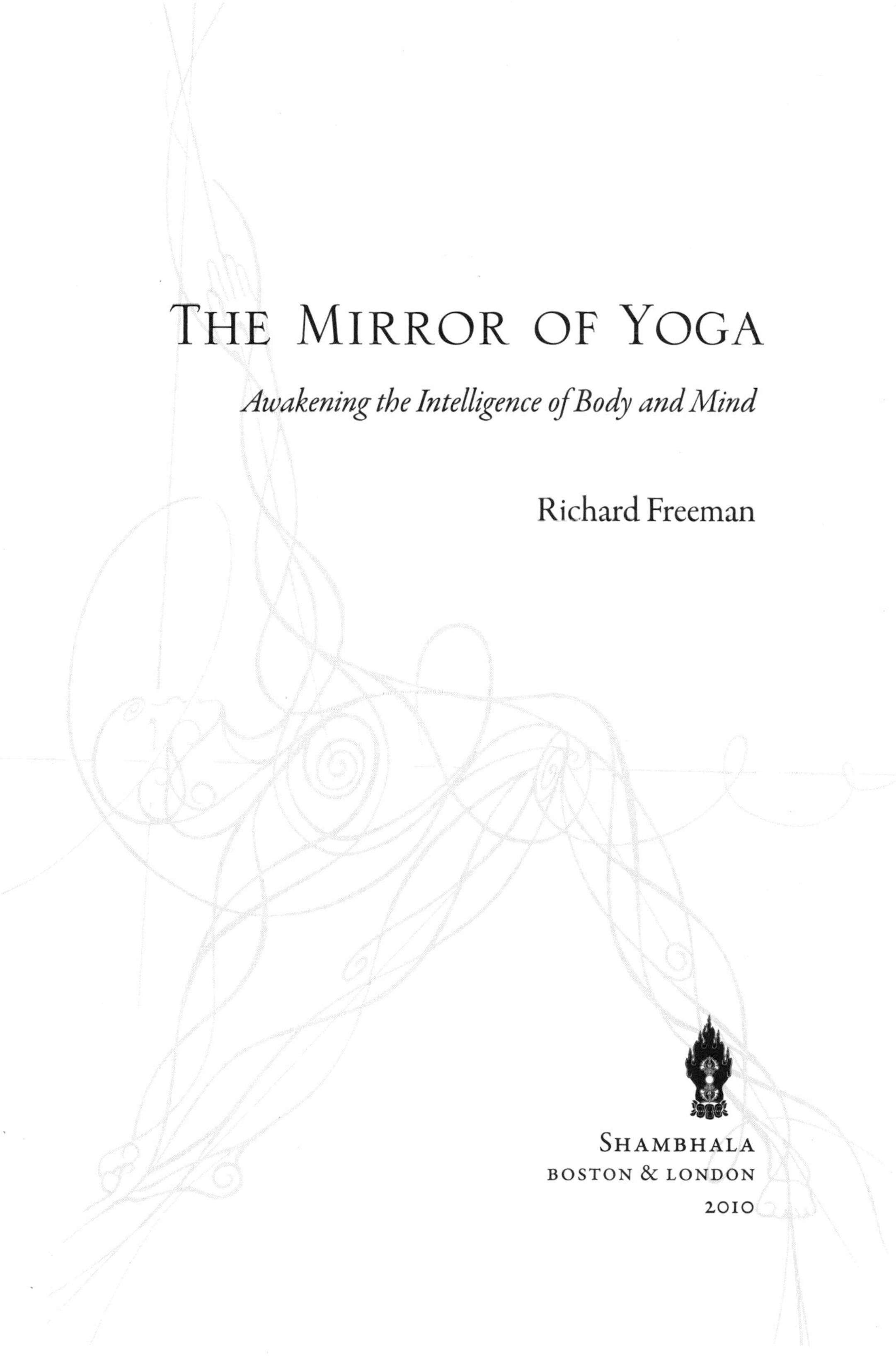

The Mirror of Yoga

Awakening the Intelligence of Body and Mind

Richard Freeman

Shambhala
Boston & London
2010

Shambhala Publications, Inc.
Horticultural Hall
300 Massachusetts Avenue
Boston, Massachusetts 02115
www.shambhala.com

9 8 7 6 5 4 3 2 1

First Edition
Printed in the United States of America

♾This edition is printed on acid-free paper that meets the American National Standards Institute z39.48 Standard.
♻This book was printed on 30% postconsumer recycled paper. For more information please visit www.shambhala.com.

Distributed in the United States by Random House, Inc., and in Canada by Random House of Canada Ltd

Designed by Gopa & Ted2, Inc.

Freeman, Richard, 1950–
The mirror of yoga: awakening the intelligence of body and mind / Richard Freeman. — 1st ed.
p. cm.
Includes index.
ISBN 978-1-59030-795-3 (hardcover: alk. paper)
1. Yoga. I. Title.
BL1238.52.F74 2010
613.7'046—dc22
2010006461

In loving memory

Sri. K. Pattabhi Jois, Guruji

1915–2009

Contents

Introduction

Yoga begins with listening. When we listen, we are giving space to what is. We are allowing other people to be what they are, and we are sanctioning our own bodies and our own minds to fully manifest. Yoga also begins in the present moment. Many classic texts, such as the *Yoga Sūtra* by Patañjali, start with the word *atha*, meaning "now," which refers to this very notion. In the context of the *Yoga Sūtra*, the use of the word *atha* means that we have come to a point in our lives where we are ready to wake up from our conditioned existence and our habitual ways of behaving, thinking, and interacting with the world. It insinuates that we are finally ready to get real and to discover the essence of all existence that lies deep down in the core of our own heart and at the center of our being. It is from this experience of the root of life in the present moment that a yoga practice can actually be generated. Patañjali's use of the word *now* implies that we have most likely tried many, many other things in order to wake up and to find happiness. We have probably pursued all different types of pleasures, and perhaps we have explored various philosophical teachings and disciplines and maybe even religious practices in order to give life meaning. But still, something is not quite right. When all of our attempts to find meaning are seen to have been inadequate for the job, then we come into our present situation and *this* is where the practice of yoga truly begins—right here, right now.

Yoga is freedom. It is freedom from the fear of not knowing who we are, from presenting a face to the world that is not truly representative of who we feel ourselves to be, and from pretending to believe in things that we do not really know to be true. This is the liberation we find in yoga as we return to the present moment: to our natural mind and to a state of complete happiness. It is unlikely we are drawn to yoga in a conscious search for this freedom, but rather that we find yoga attractive because we imagine that it will make us happy, and there are many ideas about what happiness is that may invite us in. We may begin our practice to benefit the body; to become healthy, strong, flexible, sexy, or vibrant. We may see yoga on a more superficial level as simply an answer to our boredom or as a good way to meet people. Then one day in a yoga class we may experience the mind spontaneously dropping into a state of calm and clarity, a feeling that draws us back again in search of that natural sense of balance. The particulars of why we come to yoga may take on any number of forms, and all of them are honorable starting points for the practice because each doorway that reveals itself is a path into the deep matrix of what yoga truly is, and each entrance reveals that ultimately we have come in search of the mystical experience—a timeless sense of complete freedom and happiness.

Whatever reason brings us to yoga, it is imperative to start from exactly where we actually are, and this requires at least a moment of true honesty. It necessitates that we remove all facades; that we give up pretending to know things that we do not actually know; and that we remove the veils of denial and deception we have draped over the real condition of our circumstance, our mind, and our heart. No matter what your motivation for beginning a practice—even if it is embarrassingly neurotic or selfish—if you can simply see the reality of that motivation, then you have found the proper place for beginning your own practice. Indeed, the ground upon which you are standing as you dive in is the only way to begin a genuine yoga practice. When you can see and accept things as they are, no matter how distorted your idea about what yoga might be or what it might do for you, then everything starts to become quite interesting. Because you have come to the source of all things—the fountainhead, the wish-fulfilling tree of yoga—you will get far more than you ever imagined possible.

As we work through this book we will explore the profound and mysterious depths of yoga that lie underneath the wide variety of practices and beliefs that are normally associated with it. We will touch on various traditional philosophies that are used as tools in yoga, and we will examine a variety of physical and mental exercises that are parts of the practice of yoga. Through this book we hope to inspire the intelligence, imagination, and heart to open into direct experience, free of philosophy and technique, so that we can simply be here whole and happy.

The Mirror of Yoga

1

Phases of the Practice and Classical Forms of Yoga

There are many different styles of yoga practice: diverse methodologies, and distinct lineages. Though there is no single yoga philosophy, no one methodology, there *is* an underlying web of similarity that connects all approaches to yoga, and it is this deeply woven interconnectedness—the matrix within the pattern of what we call yoga—that we are going to be exploring in this book. By examining and illuminating different types of practices, philosophies, and methodologies, and by finding the pattern of interconnectedness that lies beneath them, the essence of yoga is revealed and we can truly be who we are.

Well known for spectacular physical poses, haṭha yoga is actually a system of working the body and breath in order to investigate meditatively deep and subtle feelings, responses, and reflexes in relation to the conditioning of the mind. Insight into the subtle nature of sensation and its relationship to internal breathing patterns is believed to be the key to insight into the true nature of the mind. *Haṭha* means "sun" (*ha*) and "moon" (*tha*), and it can be used to describe any yoga practice that unites opposite patterns within the nervous system in order to open up the core of the body for our observation. A central component of haṭha yoga is āsana, or the practice of yoga postures, in which we work the body; we turn it, twist it, stretch it, and explore its subtleties. Another component is prāṇāyāma, in which we stretch, unfold, refine, and closely observe the breathing. Within these physical practices of haṭha yoga we work the body like we knead dough when making bread, so that it becomes transformed from an amorphous lump of unconscious flesh and bones into something that is vital and full of life. Through this work we find that both the body and the mind begin to wake up; they begin to unite with each other and with our everyday experience of life. As we continue to practice we gradually begin to find that we can extract from the body all of the juice of insight and consciousness that lies within it.

Another type of yoga is jñāna yoga, which focuses on the intelligence and our ability to deeply inquire into the nature of things. *Jñāna* means "knowing" or "wisdom." It is an infinitely refined search into the way the mind works, in combination with how perception and feelings work. It is the yoga of insight into the actual nature of our mind and reality. In jñāna yoga we foster the capacity to discriminate very precisely between that which is true, eternal, joyous, and that which is completely impermanent, superficial, and even delusionary. There are many approaches to jñāna yoga, some teaching instant enlightenment as a leap of understanding into the meaning of life. In this form you have a flash of insight into the meaning of reality, and from that moment on the mind has begun to wake up in such a way that life is merely a continuous unfolding insight. The experience of this form of jñāna yoga is something like when you finally get a joke and there is a sense of comprehension, relief, insight—the "aha!" feeling. Other jñāna yoga schools teach a gradual awakening, applying over time a more rigorous path, a complete study of everything, as a means of recognizing underlying patterns of perception and mind so that the true nature of the self—the true nature of the universe—is revealed. Still other jñāna yoga schools teach both an instant and a gradual awakening, based on how the mind is framing the very questions of time, existence, self, and consciousness. Any approach to jñāna yoga must eventually turn its fine intelligence back on itself to undo all sense of false ego and pride that a practitioner might take in their own partial understanding.

Aṣṭāṅga yoga, though familiar to some as strictly a series of postures accompanied by specific patterns of breathing and gazing, is actually the broad system of yoga that forms the context for posture and breathing practices. *Aṣṭāṅga* means "eight limbs," implying that there are many different interrelated approaches within this school that are used to develop a laserlike focus of the mind. This focus is utilized to explore any and all physical and mental phenomena that arise in order to reveal that they are composites of their backgrounds and not anything separate or eternal. This revelation or insight leads the aṣṭāṅga practitioner on and on to deeper states of insight into the nature of their mind and the world, and eventually to liberation from conditioned existence. The primary ground on which aṣṭāṅga yoga is built is an establishment of the ethical framework from which the other limbs of practice may then flourish. The support built from the first two limbs, the yamas and the niyamas, provides a net of interactive kindness and responsiveness to both oneself and within relationships to others. As part of the framework, the next two limbs—the physical practices of āsana (postures) and prāṇāyāma (breathing practices)—begin to open the body, the breath, and the sense fields, deconditioning the practitioner from the overlay of concepts and memories. This paves the way for the meditative limbs to work easily and with less danger of becoming lost in thought and abstracted away from the body. In the fifth limb, pratyāhāra, the mind is trained to observe the sense fields without identifying with or separating objects from their background. In this way the attention no longer moves about in the sense fields. In the sixth limb, dhāraṇā, the attention is concentrated on a single area. The seventh limb, dhyāna, occurs when concentration flows without conflict or tension. In the eighth limb, samādhi, the mental habit of making a constructed object and subject stops. This allows a free, unobstructed view of whatever is being observed, allowing insight into its true nature. The advantage of aṣṭāṅga yoga's multiple approaches through various limbs is that it ensures that practitioners do not neglect any aspect of their inner or outer life, and this in turn fosters the ability to stay grounded in reality rather than being swept away by concepts or fantasy.

Bhakti—the yoga of love and devotion—is another type of yoga in which deep emotion and the primacy of relationship to others and to God are cultivated and examined. Any selfishness arising from a misperception of oneself or the other gradually burns away. Through the bhakti practice, emotions become experienced as essential components of devotion, and they are channeled into ecstatic sensation. Some schools of bhakti have a conception of the beloved as a divine person, while others prefer an open view of the ultimate nature of God, one's self, and others. The practice of bhakti often includes chanting and visualization, which allow us to viscerally experience a sense of connectedness to the real nature of the other, to God, and to the joyous nature of all things. A state of mind that is open to experiencing whatever is arising as being connected to the beloved (or as being the beloved itself) removes the conditioned overlays of emotion, thought, preconception, and other functions of mind that normally distract and distort reality.

All over the world the schools of tantra have captured attention and interest, often because they are erroneously associated only with their aspects that deal with sexuality. But there is much more to tantric yoga. The word *tantra* actually means a thread or a weaving of threads, and in the context of yoga this refers to the idea of weaving a net of intelligence within, through, and beyond the body and mind. Tantric yoga is considered by some to be a subset of haṭha yoga, and others would say that haṭha yoga is a specific set of techniques within tantric practice. In fact tantra and haṭha yoga alike are organized around the principle that all things are sacred. Many yoga practices are designed to unplug the normally closed central channel of the body, the suṣumnā nāḍī, which extends from the center of the pelvic floor right up through the crown of the head and which is considered to be the most sacred channel of awareness within the body. Within tantra, which is particularly focused on the sacred nature of everything, deep attention is given to the fine details of all types of experience as a means of reorganizing and balancing the inner processing of experience around and through this central axis of the body. The tantric use of sacred sound and form within the practices has the potential to open the central axis to a flow of focused attention and deep sensation. When the concentration enters the suṣumnā nāḍī in this way, the mind automatically starts to fold in on itself, resting in ecstatic depths of insight through pure awareness. Outwardly, tantra is the practice of realizing that the ordinary world and everything we do in the world are incredibly sacred. Within tantra there are many practices that ritualize our ordinary sense perceptions and our everyday activities in the world, allowing us to eventually enter the inner realm of the suṣumnā nāḍī and become grounded in reality just as it is.

Another approach to yoga, one which helps to free us from being too esoteric and exclusive is karma yoga, the yoga of work or action. Since the nature of the body and mind, except in the deepest of trance of samādhi, is movement, we find that by sanctifying that movement—our actions and our work—the mind can be freed from attachment to the outcome or the fruit of our action. This is a potent way of eliminating the ego from daily and necessary work. Karma yoga allows all types of people to practice, even those who might not have the luxury of time or the opportunity to study the contemplative paths. It allows us to concentrate on our work, transforming it into an art and a source of satisfaction in and of itself. Perhaps the most important aspect of karma yoga is that when work is practiced as an offering to other beings or to God, awareness of others is enhanced, which in turn decreases narcissistic tendencies, making all approaches to yoga easier.

Around 600 B.C.E. Gautama (Sakyamuni) Buddha gave birth to a brilliant vision of yoga now known as Buddhism. Gautama Buddha taught the practices and philosophies of traditional yoga but rejected the authority of the then-dominant Vedic religion within the existing schools. He turned the philosophical and religious language used to talk about yoga on its head by teaching that there is no permanent self or ātman. He also stated that a belief in a separate self leads to egotism, craving, and suffering. Meditation or deep yoga practice gives a direct experience of this truth. One of the main terms for truth and consciousness within the traditional yoga language is *ātman,* and the declaration of the apparent opposite created quite a philosophical and political stir. This has led to centuries of debate among practitioners and philosophers as to what they really mean by the terms *ātman* and *no-ātman.* Buddhist and other yoga schools have been beneficial mirrors for each other, stimulating mutual growth by pointing out each other's blind spots and prodding each other into practicing rather than resting on doctrine. The Buddha's approach also helped to open the practice of yoga to all people, many of whom had been disqualified by the strict caste structure of Indian society.

There are numerous subsets of these primary schools of yoga. It is important to remember that all of the classic schools and their subsets are interrelated; they use each other's methodologies in varying proportions because no one school can accurately describe the immediate and overall process that is yoga. Explaining the whole truth, the metaphysical ground of being, nature, or God is always beset with difficulty and paradox. It is like the eye trying to see itself. Any point of view or system sees and explains things well, but all have blind spots. Others outside the system are needed to fill in the blind spots. As yoga students and teachers, we tend to become attached to and prejudiced about our own school and methodology. It is natural under most circumstances to identify with the club we belong to because there is a certain kind of security and satisfaction in that; there is also an inherent tendency of mind to want to feel that our own system is better than others—even for those who study and practice yoga. Consequently, it is not uncommon to simply rest on the superficial levels of the school we consider to be our own. In so doing, we fool ourselves into a state of pseudo-satisfaction, hiding in a simplistic understanding of the teachings and conveniently avoiding practice, which is needed in order to understand deeply. It is safe and comfortable on the surface because going deeply requires that we question the structure of everything, including the structure of the very school to which we belong.

The specific differences between traditional schools of yoga are less important than the fact that most are intended to eventually lead to a direct experience of reality. Whether they are successful depends on the intelligence, devotion, and ability of the individual students and teachers to correctly adapt and interpret teachings and practices. The most powerful traditional schools—those with long lineages that have been tossed around and refined for many generations—represent the epitome of human inquiry into reality. These schools are deeply rooted in the ancient cultures of India, dating back well over five thousand years, and each has evolved over time, some coming from still older traditions that have flowed together and merged, and others developing as traditions splintered apart. The actual history of each is complex and distinctive, and for many schools we will never really know who the formers, reformers, and innovators were. What we do know, however, is that for any school to stay alive and applicable within today's environment, it must continue to evolve. But we must beware, because an excellent, profound, living tradition of yoga can still be worn by an idiot as a decoration for his or her ego, while a sincere, open-minded, inquisitive student of a fractured lineage can breathe new life and insight into that tradition for everyone's benefit.

The Vedas are the ancient hymns with which many of the religions, customs, and myths of India are intertwined. These beautiful and lengthy hymns have been memorized and passed down in the families of Vedic Brāhmaṇa priests for at least five millennia and, until recently, remained strictly an oral tradition. Over time the Vedas evolved in a rich crossroad of ancient cultures, mysticism, shamanism, and religion. Mysterious, complex, brilliant, and somewhat inscrutable in their poetry, they are believed to be a timeless revelation of truth and are sometimes used by their followers as an ultimate authority. Some schools of yoga claim that their own interpretations are direct revelations of the Vedas and are therefore the only true teachings. The arcane nature of the hymns, however, always leaves their meaning open to interpretation, and this has been helpful in the evolution of yoga practice and philosophy. Many of the early strands of yoga practice contributed to and were influenced by the formation of the Vedas, and yet other schools claimed that yoga evolved as a way to move beyond the Vedas' limited and ultimately materialist orthodox world.

Following the Vedas historically, around 800 B.C.E., there appeared the early Upaniṣads and other scriptures, which began a new age of direct philosophical inquiry and systematic, deliberate investigation into yogic practice and experience. Then over time came epic poems, such as the *Mahābhārata* and the *Rāmāyaṇa*, the Purānas or histories, the sūtras of the different schools, the tantras, the haṭha yoga texts, the ongoing creation of new Upaniṣads, the Buddhist canon are just a few of the thousands of scriptures that followed the Vedas and relate directly or indirectly to yoga in some form. All major schools of yoga have classical texts or scriptures associated with them; many traditions share some of the same texts. These texts are generally written in Sanskrit or one of its derivatives, such as Pālī. Occasionally texts were written in a local dialect, making them more accessible to contemporary students who lived within the area.

The Sanskrit language, in which many but not all of the classic texts were written, has developed a special status. The word *Sanskrit* means "perfect," "polished," or "constructed," and as a language it has been refined in this manner since its first use in the early Vedic hymns. It has been crafted to reveal the refined sound and resonance that easily form mantras; the method of joining one word to the next allows a continuation of a base meditative resonance into which the attention is magnetically drawn. In fact, the experience of chanting itself is considered to be an experience of a yogic state. As was true with the teachings from many ancient cultures, Sanskrit hymns were often composed in verse or in a meter with rhyme so that they were easily memorized and could be chanted as a means of passing teachings from generation to generation. To this day the memorization and chanting of traditional Sanskrit texts is considered a sacred practice in India, and it continues to enrich a cultural connection to ancient yogic philosophy because the contemplation of a text as it is chanted naturally sows seeds of insight, which result in application of the message of the text. Classical yogic traditions are the result of hundreds of thousands of people over many generations reflecting on the way their minds work as they investigate their own immediate experience of reality. A wonderful aspect of teachings from an ancient tradition is the natural enrichment of ideas that occurs in this process. With so much practice, experimentation, reflection, and communication, individuals and entire schools evolve. Over time real communication and translation between the practitioners of different schools happens naturally, which refines everyone's technique, language, and breadth of understanding. The universal or common patterns of a practice and its supporting teachings are exposed, renewed, and clarified by the often-uncomfortable exposure to others outside the group.

The purpose of this book is not to make you a premature eclectic. It is not to confuse you with the great variety of yoga philosophies, traditions, and practices you may encounter, nor is it to make you into an armchair enlightened being. Instead it is to allow all of us to slow down a bit so that we can delve deeply into the subject rather than skidding along on the surface side to side, from one school back to another. We are aiming at the core of the teachings. By sticking with it and going deeply we find that the jewel at the heart of every valid school is that we are eventually invited to face ourselves just as we face reality. There is a wonderful story about a man digging a well. He would begin digging down and after five or six feet of digging, which is very hard work, he would find no water, and so he would climb out of the little hole he had made, move twenty feet over, and dig another hole for his well. But after digging about six feet down, he would give up again, move twenty feet in another direction and start digging again. This went on, and on, and on, and he never found water. So it is with the restless ego pursuing yoga, seeking ornaments for an improved self-image and new ways of feeling better, but avoiding the true facts of life. When the school or practice becomes difficult—which is precisely the entry point into reality—it is at *this* crisis point that you really have to drop your pretenses and keep digging deeper into the experience. However, all too often it is right at this juncture that we tend to give up the practice. We move on to a "better" teacher or a "more interesting" school, rather than sticking with it and investigating the inner work that is the purpose of the school and the teachings in the first place. Of course if the teacher (or school) has not done his or her work of sticking with the practice at the point of difficulty, then it could be time to find a different teacher, and this discriminative awareness—knowing when to stick with it and when to move on—is part of what a good yoga practice teaches.

Most traditions of yoga are designed to inspire us to dig a deep well from precisely where we are within our own unique circumstances. By digging deeply we come across a direct experience of what is happening right here, right now. In that begins an awakening into the actual nature of pure consciousness and the function of mind. There is a taste of complete liberation and release. Letting go of the urge to compulsively search for freedom, we become unshackled from identification with the impermanent forms of the world. We no longer associate ourselves with the body and the self-image, and this enables us to appreciate ourselves and the whole natural world in a completely fresh way. Whatever tradition captures our mind, whatever ancient, medieval, or hybrid form of yoga we find that works for us so that we may dig deeply into the nature of the direct experience, that is the starting point. If it allows real work and authentic inquiry within our own unique circumstances, it is the tradition to follow enthusiastically. At the same time, be aware of how the ego function of the mind might turn any practice, tradition, or great starting point into an escape, a distraction, or even a political agenda. A sincere yoga practice can save us from this.

It is useful to examine the meta-pattern that occurs around any of these traditions when we finally get down to it and start digging a well. A meta-pattern is what links a form or pattern into its context and then links that context onto another layer of context. It is the universal nature of patterns that there is no absolute or final pattern. In our normal process of perception, everything we are aware of—specific objects, feelings, sensations, or thoughts—is actually a pattern, not a solid and permanent thing. Our beloved dog, the pang of sadness we feel at the loss of a friend, our definition of who we are as a teacher or a parent, or even the physical pain we feel in our neck—these are all forms that are part of our own patterns of perception. With close scrutiny we see that whatever form we perceive has underneath it other forms that do not appear. That which we identify as a complete form, one that we understand or know, is actually an expression of the complex layers that make up the whole beneath it. Our dog is an evolved domesticated animal, a specific breed or a mix of breeds, a friend, a miraculous being, and a protector, to name just a few of the layers that merge together to form the pattern in our mind of "my dog." No matter what it is we are experiencing, the form itself often conceals its background and appears as an object separate from everything else. But through continued observation and prolonged contemplation of any perceived form, we can eventually see through the form itself and recognize the context within which the form rests. Sooner or later we see that the specific form is a unique composite of the patterns that make up its background.

For instance, when we watch the water swelling in the ocean we can identify this pattern as a wave. We know the wave is not actually separate from the ocean, but until we broaden our perspective, the ocean and the wave remain two distinct forms that we identify in our mind as being separate. If we allow the mind to release so that our arbitrary boundaries of definition that separate wave from ocean may dissolve, we can easily see the union of what at first appeared to be two separate forms. Spontaneously we experience, right through the core of our being, a deep flash of insight the instant we recognize the union of those two "separate" forms. In this transformation of specific forms, the underlying nest in which every internal and external aspect of the universe rests is seen, and we experience the interconnected weave of everything. Specific superficial forms (that is, the wave) are the patterns the mind creates as a means of quickly and efficiently understanding its perceptions. But when we let our contingent forms go and experience the interconnecting meta-pattern that envelopes and penetrates those forms, our theories and formulations (even about the underlying pattern itself) are suspended and dissolve into alert, open intelligence. Connecting in this way to the present moment, the very nature of our being is revealed.

When we practice yoga, we explore this notion of the meta-pattern that envelopes and penetrates all that we perceive. Many philosophical traditions have contemplated this notion of the interconnectedness of life, and studying classic texts from most traditions gives insight into the idea. The physical nature of many traditional yoga practices gives an unusual visceral understanding of the interpenetration of all aspects of life, which can be uniquely clear and profound because it is a direct experience of the interpenetration of form and idea within our own body. As it turns out the human body, *your* body, is the ideal ground for understanding and experiencing this notion of a meta-pattern, what we might call an interlinking matrix or a yoga matrix.

In normal, everyday life our attention is projected out into the world so that we can make sense of what we perceive, allowing us to navigate quickly and easily through our experience. Typically when we look at the body we see it through those same filters and theories. We may see it as a bag of skin filled with bones and blood, or as a continuum of suffocating, painful frustration used to validate all of the miserable opinions we have of others and of ourselves. Our focus might be on just one part of the body—the image of our face, or the belly, the thighs, the nervous system, the musculature—to the exclusion of all other aspects. Through a consistent yoga practice, all the different notions we may concoct about what the body is and who we are eventually arise as objects for our meditation. When we stay with our observation, digging our well deeper and deeper, we begin to see all the way through the forms of perception we have created. Seeing through our theories *about* the body we are led into an actual experience of the core of our own body itself. We are able to look through the deep emotions and patterns that make up our subjective awareness, and we also see through those parts of ourselves that we have objectified and have identified as the body itself. We see that the ideas of skin, bones, organs, and all that we know to be the physical body are actually just the culturally agreed-upon forms that we have identified in order to comprehend the arising of the particular pattern of manifestation we call "humans." Through this practice we discover that the human body is far more than any of the theories about it. In meditation the body is experienced as an open matrix of awareness through which theories, thoughts, and sensations come and go.

This is perhaps the most refined and wonderful aspect of the yoga tradition—that through our own body we learn to understand the universe. We do this by slowing everything down, as if saying, "Wait a minute, we are going to look with fresh eyes and listen with opened ears and a renewed awareness in all of our senses at this mystery of life that is presenting itself through, within, and as the body." In this way we can temporarily suspend all judgments and conclusions about the body. Again and again, with fresh eyes, we closely examine all of our theories and patterns of experiencing what we know as the body. In this suspension we are supported by the mystery of the underlying and ultimately unknowable matrix of open intelligence. Our feelings, thoughts, sensations, and emotions reveal the interconnectedness of immediate

matrix. womb
Begging + devotion very close
that's why Bhuddah took ↑ the begging bow

experience with the whole world of underlying patterns. This process of realization happens spontaneously when we allow ourselves to fully perceive whatever we are experiencing in the moment, without becoming attached to the perception and, at the same time, without rejecting it. As we become more skillful in our yoga practice, we learn to perceive deeply without creating a "story" that we (and others) must believe to be true or false, good or bad, safe or unsafe. Eventually we do not buy into our story lines, nor do we become attached to their outcome—we do not hold on to them or reject them. We learn to become aware of our deep perceptions as both vital and real, but more important, we recognize that our own forms of perceptions are the gateway into the matrix that intimately connects us to everything else.

Matrix means the "womb." It comes from the word *mother,* and it implies that there is a nest that interconnects and sustains everything. Whatever your practice is, no matter what you think or experience, all of this is cradled within the matrix called yoga. The matrix itself has no motivation or desire, but it allows each and every *thing* within it to evolve fully so that everything finds its mate and its complement in order to become actualized. Just as a mother, with unconditional love, supports and nurtures her child, the matrix allows everything to grow, flourish, and flower, and it also allows everything to die or to disappear. In this way all things discover themselves, and they also ascertain their relationship to and their interconnectedness with everything else. From whatever point we initiate our own yoga practice—and incidentally, we must begin from where we actually are—this matrix starts to open for us, and we find that we can go ever deeper into our own immediate experience, just as when digging a well. We see that each philosophical stance and every practice is a composite of all other philosophical perspectives and of all the other types of practice. We experience for ourselves that each is nested within a more complex interwoven pattern of the yoga matrix, where no type of practice or theory is dominant and where the pure radiant presence, the underlying nature of the matrix itself, is revealed.

When we experience this process of insight we see not only the interconnectedness but also the temporary or impermanent nature of whatever appears to us. Eventually this realization comes to include our own bodies and the bodies of all those we love. Understanding viscerally as well as intellectually that everything is impermanent is terrifying to the ego structure. A great deal of clinging, remorse, and avoidance naturally arises in the face of this reality. But with close meditative observation of such strong emotions, by watching states of dread and theories of doom and oblivion that surface, they too are seen to open up into their contexts. In this way the background of unconditional love and absolute support that is the true nature of an open mind is revealed. This awareness allows us to be at peace, even in the face of impermanence, and it also fosters a sense of love for others in spite of the fact that we might not know them perfectly well. We might not understand others or be able to control them, we might not even like them, but we can still have unconditional love for them. Likewise, this deep visceral understanding of the interconnectedness of all things allows us to accept the world in all of its multiplicity and complexity, without constantly analyzing and inserting our ego into the situation. We experience that the entire universe as it is being given to us in this moment is a great joyous being whose essence is pure consciousness.

This may sound a little idealistic and perhaps even unattainable, however it is actually quite straightforward, and it happens automatically by deeply observing what *is* as it arises. Through our yoga practice we learn to cultivate this observational skill, seeing what is immediately before us, so that eventually the practice transforms into something that penetrates every aspect of life. We hone the skill of focusing the mind on whatever pattern of perception it lights upon; whatever we are thinking, feeling, sensing, emoting becomes the object of meditation. By paying attention to the pattern of whatever is happening right now—and it could be a pattern we would normally consider to be miserable or neurotic or even ecstatic—by allowing the mind to rest *there* we find a gateway into understanding the whole beneath it. Through this meditative approach the context of that which we are observing is revealed, and quite easily, without a sense of anxiety, we perceive the background as an interlinking web of pure consciousness that has manifested as whatever we are observing. It becomes clear that the one point that appeared so separate within our attention is actually interpenetrating its immediate background, and that this same background (that also could be perceived as separate) melts into its own background, and so on. We experience this in a deeply physical, embodied way when the practice of yoga postures is done well. A viscerally grounded understanding of interconnectedness prompts the mind to soak deeper and deeper through various layers of background to where our perceptions and even sensations appear to us as sacred, inexplicable, and wonderful.

When we are able to appreciate the content of our mind in this way, whether it is perfect or imperfect, we have temporarily suspended the habit of reducing our immediate experience to theories about it. Just as when we look at the tip of an iceberg and intuit that it is a vast chunk of ice with a massive bottom section that is hidden to us, so too we can distinguish the deep matrix of yoga as ever new and always sacred through the tip of our own perceptions, which are revealed through the practices and through the immediate world as it appears before us. We realize, too, that neither of these perspectives (the top of the iceberg or what lies beneath it) is better than the other, nor is one possible without the other. Through a consistent yoga practice we gradually learn to switch easily between seeing points of view—the specific and the universal perspective of our experience. This fluidity of viewpoint allows for a depth and richness of understanding far greater than any one perspective might ever offer. Simultaneously seeing things from both a global and specific perspective sounds more difficult than it is. Imagine a forest thick with trees. If you are next to any particular tree you have a unique viewpoint of the whole forest. The nature of the forest is that the trees hide its totality from within and that you can never see the whole complete forest when you are in it. You can fly above the forest and see it as a green, textured sea, but even this perspective is not actually complete because the details of any one point within the forest are not perceptible from so far away, so in a sense each viewpoint within the forest gives you a rich taste of "forest" that is far more vivid and real than the sense you get when you observe the entire thicket of trees from above. The essence of the taste of "forest" is mystery. What makes forests so calming and exciting to be in is that most of the viewpoints are hidden, they are mysterious to you, yet in the midst of the forest, the one viewpoint you have is astounding. As if nestled within a forest, a good yoga practice reveals a sense of safety in the insight that everything we are observing is at once specific to us alone and at the same time interconnected to the universal structure of all that is outside ourselves.

In Indian mythology the god Indra is said to have a net of illusion (maya) that he casts over beings in order to either bind or free them. The net has been called the Jeweled Net of Indra because there is a beautiful jewel at each juncture or linking point in the lattice. The metaphor of this net demonstrates that illusion and insight are two sides of the same phenomenon. When ignorance and egotism are dominant, the net falsely makes everything appear separate. In our struggle to get out of the net we grasp at sense objects, which causes us to become more and more entangled since those objects are not actually separate from everything else; they only appear to be so. If you are fortunate and are able to listen to teachings about the nature of reality and illusion, you are able to look closely at the net itself. If this is the case, once the net is cast over you and you come to an intersection in the mesh and look into the facets of the jewel you find there, you are able to see all the other junctures and the thousands of jewels within the net. The entire pattern of the net of Indra is contained in each point or jewel. Seeing this kindles the understanding that from any point of view the truth of all experience and existence can be discovered. At the same time you

Jeweled Net of Indra (1)

The Jeweled Net of Indra represents the way we might experience the universe when the intelligence is purified. At each intersection of the net there is a jewel, and each facet of the jewel reflects all of the other jewels of the net. This is a universe in which each point is the center, and in which we find the whole universe within each point. When viewed this way, there is no longer the illusion of a separate self and we cease trying to escape. Seeing that every "thing" is a composite of its background, wherever the mind goes, that very place is the supreme place. There is no inside and no outside to the net, and there is no one center and no supreme point of view. Every center and each point of view contains all of the other centers and points of view.

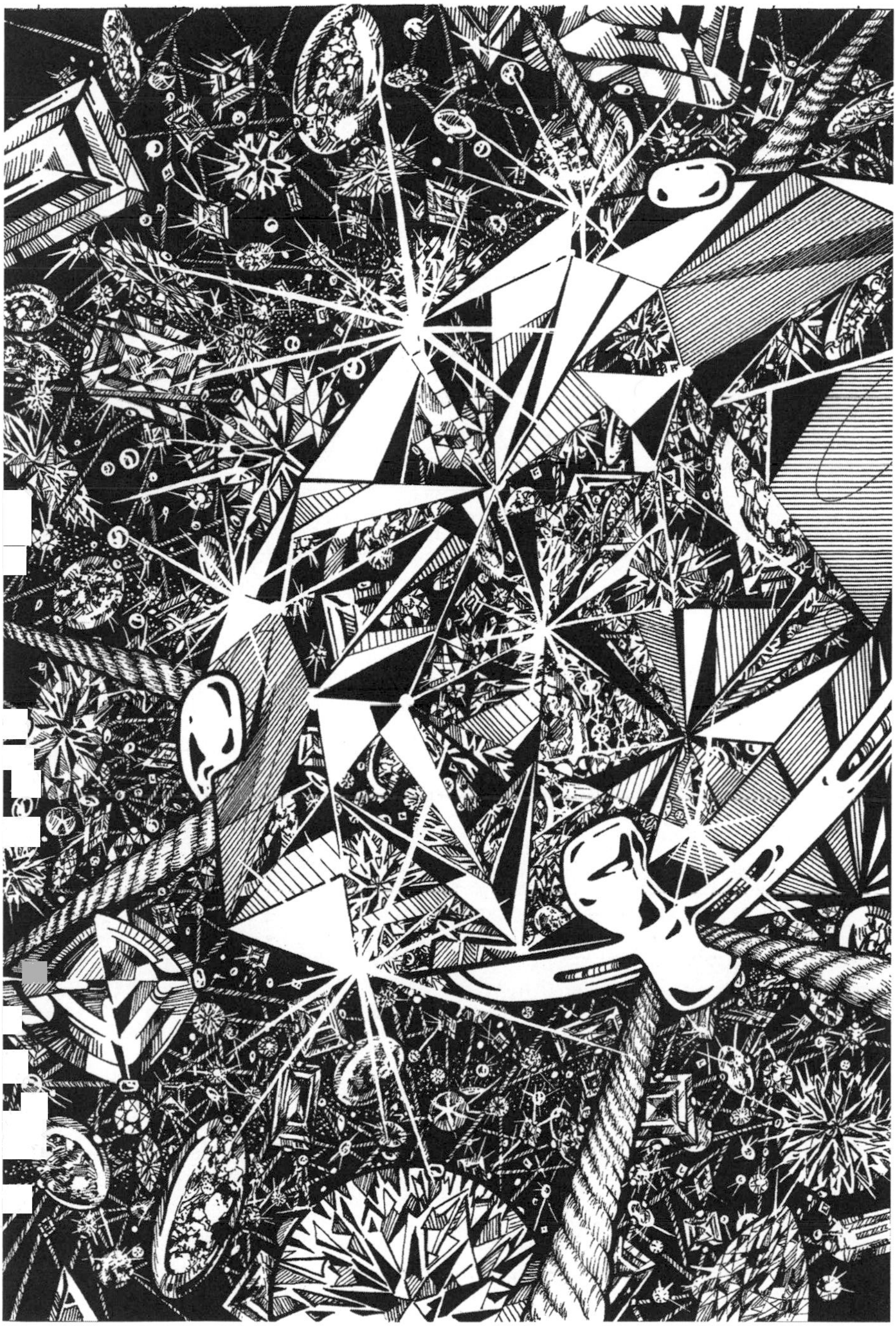

can see that the appearance of things as separate forms is an illusion, and you realize that escaping from your place, your viewpoint within the net, is unnecessary; instead you become wise to it, you see through your own illusions. Likewise the yoga practice reveals a jeweled net of perception within our own experience. During the practice, wherever your mind goes, if you make that perception—like a jewel within the net—the object of your meditation, then your awareness is automatically transformed into a seed of insight that reflects deeper forms of consciousness and compassion contained within the entire net of your immediate experience. Through the observation of your own senses the insight that every point contains in it, as its background, everything else becomes crystal clear. If you meditate on whatever is arising in this way, a sense of immense pleasure and satisfaction starts to flood your awareness and you find that it is as if you are living in a continually self-renewing, open, magical, and fresh experience of pure life. Your perception of the simplest sensation or the most ordinary everyday experience can take you to unlimited depth, and this is truly where the heart of yoga is revealed.

Dissolving in this way into the heart of yoga is an act of honesty. It is the art of humility and of genuine awe and appreciation for the life process as it is. Yoga reveals itself when we allow our senses, our intelligence, and our bodies to unfold free of a self-image or any sort of goal or motivation. Through this process of openness and expansion, we find ourselves engulfed in a rare form of freedom in which we experience the luminosity of each jewel of our awareness increase as it reflects upon every other gem within the net of our own consciousness. The more we meditate on this interpenetrating pattern, the more accessible and friendly the mystery of its interconnectedness and depth becomes, which allows us to let go and to relax, knowing that we are supported by an incredibly ancient, self-renewing latticework of tradition. We can lie back in this hammock of the matrix that is yoga, and allow reality to unfold without the distraction of any overlay of our own preconceptions and without the encumbrance of our own desires—it unfolds free and unobstructed.

2

The Body and Mind as Fields of Experience

maṇi bhrātphaṇā sahasravighṛtaviśvaṁ
bharāmaṇḍalāyānantāya nāgarājāya namaḥ
Salutations to the king of the Nagas,
to the infinite, to the bearer of the maṇḍala,
who spreads out the universe with thousands
of hooded heads, set with blazing, effulgent jewels.

The mythological serpent king Nāgarāja, the object of the mantra that serves as an epigraph to this chapter, is said to have one tail and an infinite number of heads, and is envisioned as the supporting background energy of all the things that manifest within creation. The earth that your house sits on, the foundation of the house, the floor beneath your table, the glass holding the water you are drinking, and so on, until you find something that does not serve another—all of these things are aspects of this serpent. Anything that supports, renders service, and seems to exist selflessly for another would qualify as the king of serpents. The awakened inner breath, within which the adept yogi's mind rests, is considered to be an aspect of this same expanding serpent energy. In relation to yoga practice, those things that support and assist the body of the practitioner are also looked upon and experienced as Nāgarāja. Tradition invites you to look at your practice space, your sticky mat, your block, your strap, or your sitting cushion as being manifestations of this divine serpent, and in that light, the Nāgarāja chant is used as a way to sanctify the space and the ground upon which yoga āsana are to be practiced.

We often begin yoga by chanting, which can set the correct context for the entire practice, especially if we contemplate the meaning of the words of the particular chant. In addition, the physical act of chanting can awaken the internal yoga processes by smoothly linking together the inhale and the exhale. The vibration of the chant also stimulates internal awareness as the sounds automatically bounce off of the palate in the mouth, resonating within the skull and reverberating throughout the core of the entire body. These vibratory feelings are considered to be fundamental aspects of the practice of chanting. Many chants, therefore, begin and/or end with the sound of *oṁ,* which reverberates easily as it trails off into the relaxing tone "mmm." The sound of *oṁ* travels forward and then back through the mouth along the entire palate, moving through the complete spectrum of possibilities for vowel sounds. As it flows from the lips back through the mouth, it travels behind the soft palate, where the vibration naturally ends at the upper back vault of the sinuses under the pituitary gland. The ending point of the vibration is called the *bindu,* which is translated as "droplet." The tapering off of the "mmm" sound is called the *anusvāra,* which means "extension of flow." In Indian thought, the bindu of the anusvāra is considered to be a source of a delightful nectar that when stimulated can drip down and saturate all our perceptions and experience. The physical feeling of connecting to the anusvāra is very close to what is experienced as the ending point of a good yoga practice. As we chant we find that the tapering off of the sound of the anusvāra automatically draws us into a feeling of kindness and compassion, and we discover that this same ending point of the chant is also considered to be the starting point of a yoga practice. The feeling of connecting to this point of nectar is similar to what you might experience when you have something wonderful to eat, or when you experience something delightful that resonates deeply within you and that feels in tune with your own sense of aesthetic; it is quite natural to nearly swoon with a sensation of "mmmmm" when our aesthetic sense is satisfied. Chanting creates resonance and deep sensations throughout the entire body, and these sensations facilitate the initial sense of awe and release we experience when we perceive the interconnected meta-pattern linking our immediate experience to its background. If we allow ourselves to merge into the sensations that chanting can awaken within the body, then we can begin our yoga and meditation practices within a context of intelligence and kindness. With this initial satisfaction, our individual desires and needs begin to dissipate and every object of awareness becomes a starting point for our practice.

To be honest, we often begin our study of yoga with a desire to alleviate our suffering or to find happiness or just to get a little pleasure. We may come to the practice to relax, or because our back is out of alignment, we feel frustrated, our knee hurts, or we just want a distraction. As we continue, however, our reasons for returning to yoga begin to change. We find that the practice solves our initial problems—the desires that brought us to the practice in the first place—but then deeper problems, desires, and aspirations that appear to be linked together in a chain of preferences begin to reveal themselves. "Well, at first I'm going to deal with this, then I'll get around to that, and then to this . . ." until we finally realize that although we use our body to experience the yoga, the purpose of the practice is not to cure our ills or to meet our desires, nor is it about relaxation or stimulation. In spite of the fact that yoga may temporarily delay the onset of the inevitable decay of the body, it is not ultimately about healing the body any more than it is about making us beautiful or getting rid of the body once we understand it to be an impermanent bag of skin and sensations. Instead yoga is a path to undo the root of all types of misery through the direct experience of deep, clear, open awareness. Ultimately we find that it is an attraction to the joy of this liberating experience that underlies all our other desires and that attracts us into the realm of practice in the first place.

Within the yoga tradition the body is identified as our means of practice, our instrument of perception, and our medium for perceiving reality; we know the world through our bodies. Our situation as embodied beings is astonishing. Within our individual experience we have an extremely limited point of view on the world as a whole. Each of us is located in a specific geographic location, at this one particular instant of history, and we are taking in and processing information through our eyes, ears, skin, nose, and mouth. It may seem as though we are witnessing a great deal, but in reality we have only a miniscule perspective within the vastness of the world as a whole. We arrange the information we gather so that it makes sense to us, concocting conclusions, deducing theories, and imagining all sorts of things in an attempt to understand the world, to form ideas of who we and others are, and to postulate how these aspects of the universe are related. All of this is naturally—most often unconsciously—taking place for each of us within our own body all the time, as part of the body experience. Through the practice of haṭha yoga āsana and prāṇāyāma, which focus on joining currents of opposite patterns within the body, we begin to recognize this phenomenal body as the foundation for our entire experience. This mere, mortal clump is the field of our direct experience of the world. From subtle feeling to spatial projection, we mentally project and experience past, present, and future events, beings, and worlds both near and far. As we arrange and move the body intelligently within yoga postures, the feelings, sensations, thoughts, and emotions that arise become the platform for our practice, and their intricate, impermanent patterns and details draw the attention into natural, deep meditation. There is a famous verse found in the *Tejo Bindu Upaniṣad* that says that a true yoga posture occurs when meditation flows ceaselessly and spontaneously, implying that yoga āsanas encourage an integration of body and mind. An āsana practice does not torture the body physically, nor does it cause distraction to the mind; instead, āsana invites more and more refinement when approached internally. A mindful, concentrated quality of attention is used to create a dynamic, aligned form, and the same focus of mind is used to observe the subtleties that arise throughout the body. A certain level of meditation gives rise to the posture, and a refined posture reciprocates by giving birth to an easy flow of meditation. This concentrated work of going back and forth between opposite patterns of perception, technique, and evaluation within the body and mind, and then uniting and squeezing these opposites together, produces a rich juice from the practice. Just as when you squeeze an orange you get a liquid of a vibrant color, a healthy drink, a great smell, and a delicious aesthetic absorption, so too in a yoga āsana the effect is a deep and multifaceted "juice" of experience. Within the context of a haṭha yoga practice it is the powerful juice or elixir of wisdom—insight into the true nature of the body—that we squeeze out of the physical body.

An interesting parallel to this experience inspired through a good yoga practice was the squeezing of the divine soma plant for the ancient Vedic sacrifice. The word *soma* in Sanskrit refers to an elixir or nectar. (Coincidentally, *soma* in Greek means "body.") The elixir soma was a drug with a strong psychoactive or hallucinogenic effect. After it was cleaned, cut up, and squeezed for its juice in a precise ritual, the Vedic priests would indulge in the drink. The effect must have been extraordinary. Entire chapters of the Vedic hymns, particularly the ninth chapter of the Ṛg Veda, extol the power and the ecstasy brought on by imbibing the juices of the plant. Today no one is sure of the identity of this sacred plant; that is, which psychoactive plant or mushroom soma is, though it grew at higher elevations. In the Vedic hymns and throughout Indian mythology, soma is considered to be nectar; all the gods, goddesses, and sages praised and sought soma. After drinking the soma (within ritual practice) one would sing the Vedic hymns, exquisite in their psychedelic imagery and their rich, rhythmical poetic form. The compositions were recited in an enchanting, deep, resonant, Vedic Sanskrit. Chanting the hymns is considered by the orthodoxy to be a form of yoga practice in and of itself because the act of chanting leaves the chanter mentally exhilarated, concentrated, and alert. Chanting and focusing on the profound images that arose due to the actual depth of the ideas presented in the hymns, combined with the influence of the elixir, would have given the priests deep insight into the meaning of the texts.

Within the process of yoga we take the body, just as the Vedic priests took the sacred plant that produced the nectar of soma, and through practicing the āsanas we literally twist the body around and wring it out in order to produce the nectar or the soma of yoga, which dips us directly into an experience of the true nature of our minds, and ultimately into the nature of the universe. The superficial process of the mind is not so difficult to see; it is happening all the time: it is our conclusions, symbols, theories, our ways of understanding and dealing with the world. But in order to extract the juice and find truth, meaning, and happiness, we have to press on, dig deeper, and find the hidden process of mind that exists way down, entwined and intermeshed in the very core of our body. This unfolding of the deeper mind-body connection is precisely what happens as we practice yoga āsana.

Another important and physical aspect of yoga practice is prāṇāyāma, the breathing exercises that extend the patterns of the breath and then unravel the bonds that restrict the internal breath, the prāṇa. The notion of prāṇa encompasses far more than simply the air we breathe; it is an intelligence that organizes sensations throughout the body into patterns, and then presents those patterns of feeling and sensation to our awareness. Through the practice of bringing attention to this form of the breath known as prāṇa, we are observing the sensations that arise in the body as just vibratory sensation or prāṇa alone. We trace the ends of the breath and observe the transition from inhale to exhale and back again; we become increasingly aware of the internal movements of the patterns of prāṇa within the body. Initially the breath and then feelings and sensations become the object of our meditation. Therefore, whether your yoga practice consists exclusively of sitting meditation, chanting, āsana, or prāṇāyāma, you find that the body itself is the medium through which you can discover interconnected avenues of awareness that lead to a direct experience of insight. Within any form of the practice this insight can happen, even if only for a split second, perhaps during the end of chanting the sound of oṁ, or as we sink our feet into the earth in a yoga posture, or as we relish the end of an exhalation in prāṇāyāma. At any juncture within any of the practices we may experience a sense of resonance within the core of the body that allows the mind to dissolve into its background, ushering us into a direct experience of the here and now. The physical yoga practices, therefore, give us something to observe that is immediately accessible, tangible, broad in scope, seemingly endless, but most important, grounded in the present moment and therefore undeniably impermanent. Letting go into whatever is

experience that allows the mind to dissolve
multitude of yoga practices

arising while staying solidly grounded in our body leads us to the experience of insight, and it is for this reason that the yoga traditions cherish and respect practices involving the body. Once we enter into the matrix of yoga in this way through the body, when we have a taste of the direct experience of the nature of reality, then the mind becomes satisfied. As we continue to practice, each time dipping into this immediate starting point, we learn to trust the process of melting into the present moment more and more easily. As the mind becomes more content and increasingly able to relinquish its need to identify as permanent all of the forms we perceive, we start to intuit and actually *feel* that wherever the mind settles—whether it is a thought, a concept, a feeling, or an emotion—that particular point reflects its entire background. Just as a jewel within the net of Indra reflects the entire interconnected net, so too any point upon which the mind rests is seen as a reflection of all of the body, all of the mind, all of creation. This insight allows us once again to start the practice from where we are.

Many beginning yoga practices reveal this profound process of yoga, and it is not uncommon for someone brand-new to yoga to have a flash of insight into reality during one of their first classes. Then, of course, the insight ends as quickly and as spontaneously as it arrived, and we return to the class for years longing for that same great feeling to present itself. But like so much in yoga—and in life, for that matter—experiencing the present moment is not something you do; it is something that just happens. You "do" the practices so that when the flash of insight arises, you are awake enough to notice it. So again and again we begin the practices from precisely where we are. For example, samasthitiḥ is a yoga pose in which you simply stand with your feet together and tune into the central axis of the body. It may not even seem like a yoga pose to an outside observer, but samasthitiḥ is actually a very difficult posture to do well. *Sama* means "equal," and *sthitiḥ* means "standing." In the pose eventually we end up standing with equality, with the weight distributed evenly side to side and front to back and with the center of gravity falling as on a plumb line between the front edges of the heels. The roots of the toes are spread open, the eyes find a steady, soft gaze so that the attention is stable and spread evenly around the central, vertical axis. It is very much like standing on top of a flagpole—an actual (and not recommended) yoga practice. To maintain samasthitiḥ you have to pay very close attention to what you are doing. Your awareness must be intelligent and flexible, because within the pose as you naturally start to sway off of the plumb line within your body, you automatically begin to create compensatory muscular patterns of movement that bring you back to center. Most of the time we overcompensate; we sway in one direction and then correct with an opposite swing that requires another countercorrection, and so on. We end up oscillating around the central axis in the same way a bean plant bends side to side, spiraling around a string as it grows. The yoga postures provide a field for our attention so that we recognize and respond intelligently to the patterns that are arising. In samasthitiḥ we might observe our tendency to overcompensate, or the inability of our mind to stay focused on the posture, or the tendency of our breath to become shallow or disconnected. The specifics of our observation are less important than the fact that we learn to stay on task; observing—correcting, observing—correcting, using technique and countertechnique, and then letting them go to be there for whatever is presenting itself without the distractions of concluding, projecting, accepting, or rejecting. Observing our body as the field of the practice, we gradually begin to see interrelated processes and patterns within the mind, the body, and the breath as they occur, and this allows us to fall into a very deep state of meditation. The physical practice, whether it is something simple like samasthitiḥ, a more complex pose like an advanced back bend, or a complex breathing exercise, provides an experience through which we can recognize the body as a veritable jewel within the vast net of the entire experience of the world. The physical practices become our means of watching the process of our own natural intelligence interfacing with reality; it drifts off one way before spiraling back and curling the other way, always orbiting, circling, coming closer and closer to the ideal of uniting opposite patterns within the field of our awareness. This form of intelligence lies at the heart of all of the different yoga traditions and yoga practices, and it is reflected as a fundamental process of the body and as a basic process of life itself.

The mind also offers a vast field of experience upon which the focus of attention can rest as part of the process of gaining insight into the nature of pure being. But because we must observe our own thoughts with the mind itself, watching this particular field of experience can be quite challenging. The function of mind is to represent things, to organize, to make symbols, to put things into words and categories, and then to re-sort and reorganize. In fact, the mind lives to arrange everything noteworthy, both inside and outside of the categories it creates, and to "make sense" of it all. No matter what our thoughts, doubts, fears, theories, or images of reality might be within the endless stream of observable material, it can be a difficult task to objectively observe the field of our own mind. It is with the very mind that created the patterns, the same mind that is generally unaware of its background field of assumptions, that we must observe the patterns, the field, and the assumptions. It is like the eye trying to see itself. The ego is born from and adores this conundrum, and it thrives in the process of mind. This is because, essentially, the ego is the confusion or the knotting together that occurs between pure consciousness (which could metaphorically be considered pure, open sky) and the content of consciousness (a cloud or anything that appears in the sky). The ego is referred to as the cit-acit granthi. *Granthi* means a "knot," and *cit* means "pure consciousness, pure awareness." *Acit* means "that which is unconscious" or the raw material that springs up in the present moment—that which we are aware of. In our minds knots are created when we confuse pure consciousness with the products of our mind, and this confusion is the source of the ego, which within the yogic tradition is considered to be an imaginary sense of our separation from the fabric of the universe. On a more personal level, when we imagine ourselves to be something that has been torn away from the structure of our body or from the perceptions of our mind, when we perceive ourselves as separate from the rest of creation, then the ego eagerly pops into existence.

The ego manifests when the mind identifies our own experience as having a center or self that is unique and separate from the experienced object bur related to as subject. This mentally contsructed self is felt to be the standard of true value and happiness of our being. We find that the elusive ego is fed by a need for certainty; thus even within a well-intentioned yoga practice the ego can easily surface if we transform any aspect of the practice into a formula we know. The ego desperately wants to do this because its entire function is to reduce everything, including the whole yoga tradition, to a formula that it can grasp and know definitively in order to say, "I know it! That way I don't have to do it. I've been there, done that. What's next?" It wants to reduce the truth; it even wants to diminish God to a simple idol in order to be able to say, "I got it!" In this way the ego can reign supreme over all creation. This, of course, is a perverse extension of what the healthy, beneficial process of ego actually is, which is to give us a reference point from which to begin observation and to maintain the health of the body and mind in relationship with the environment. But with the blink of an eye, the distorted ego is ready to lord over the body, the mind, all others, and eventually all of creation, which is the ultimate goal of every ego run amuck and which, as history has shown us time and again, can become a bit of a problem.

So within our yoga practice, again and again we have to make a compassionate offering into the intelligence of our very own ego. We have to practice in such a way that we allow insight into the union of the body and mind, the inhale and the exhale, the twist and the countertwist, so that we experience our own merging into what we naturally perceive as our background—all that we see as separate from ourselves. Our ego exists because we can separate from our background, and our practice becomes a constant offering of the sacred knot of the ego back into its root within the body and mind so that it can relax, calm down, and allow our natural intelligence to surface. The knot that ties selfhood to what has no selfhood, the bond that confounds pure consciousness with the unconscious, begins to unravel. But this is a very complex and slippery aspect of the practice to maintain because the mind and the ego are both so eager and endlessly willing to jump in, organize, categorize, and to "know" in order to move on. For example, the body is much, much more than the theories and maps that the mind and ego are prone to make about it. Our theories, the patterns we know as the body, are helpful to a point, but they must be released lest they turn into knots and we become stuck in the ways that we move, think, or interact with the world. It is important to understand and categorize, but it is equally important to let go of these organizational tools at the right moment. Just as we all know when we look at a map that it is not actually the territory it represents, so too we know the work of our mind and ego is not the whole picture. Maps are extremely helpful; without them you could be lost, but no map can describe the entire territory. Imagine that you were able to create the perfect map. If you had such a map it would contain everything; all of the roads, the streets, the hills, and the valleys. In fact, the perfect map would not only be a street map, but it would also be topological and would eventually be as detailed and as mysterious as the configurations of the grains of sand within the territory itself. You would have the world's perfect map, but you would not be able to fold it up and put it in your glove box, so it would be very difficult to use. That is the inherent problem with maps—they are wonderful and useful, but no map is the territory it represents. By the same token, yoga is not a quest for omnipotence as the ego would have us believe. Rather it is freedom from this never-ending, forever incomplete mission of the ego in search of omnipotence. Paradoxically, the path to this freedom lies in being able to map out a theoretical route to knowledge, power, and interrelationship with our environement, which is then dissolved before creating another map again and again, on to ever-more subtle levels of understanding.

The nature of all practice—āsana, prāṇāyāma, meditation, or the study of philosophy—is that of framing and reframing. It is a dialectical process that enables us to experience the universal nature or the meta-pattern of whatever we are observing through the practice. Stepping back we can see that the practice is both an observation of what is arising and then a letting go of the frame we were looking through. This way practice takes us deeper as we stick with it down into a closer and closer look at the basic nature of what the object is. That basic nature is one of an interconnected fullness, an openness that is the nature of pure awareness itself. Ultimately this is what all of the yoga practices do; they open up the core of our body and our heart, the roots of our navel, and the inner workings of our mind, to that which is hidden deep down inside, the true inner soma, which gives insight into the true nature of being. That insight comes about by drawing a circle and erasing a circle, by framing the object for observation then stepping back and reframing it. This is similar to what anyone does when just mulling over a problem, but it is more penetrating and focused. At some point we drop the making of a frame of any kind, and the object itself just shines out as it is, without any conceptual covers or practices involved. Whenever we practice yoga we quickly run into a paradox. This is that our mantra, our idea of God, our sacred space, our complete system, our one-pointed devotion to or concentration on anything cannot contain itself. The method, the object, the frame is useful for concentration; it is contingent, a temporary tool of convenience, but it cannot frame itself and so becomes an obstacle, like a little ego or idol that in turn needs to be seen through. Imagine you were plagued by plastic bags (symbolic of too many concepts, categories, and techniques) littering your house, so you decided to pick them up by stuffing them all into one large plastic bag. Then you still have a plastic bag. What do you do with it? Ask yourself these questions the next time you are stuffing plastic bags into a plastic bag: "Is this plastic bag the bag of all plastic bags? How do I stuff it into itself? Can it contain itself?"

We encounter this kind of self-reference paradox whenever we start to cling to any one formula within our mind, or if we hold on to any single technique within our practice (allowing the ego a special relationship to it). Paradox presents itself because eventually we discover that our idea or the technique is not complete, and that another viewpoint is arising in the background. There is great opportunity for insight whenever paradox arises; encountering one is considered to be a very auspicious, though not always comfortable, sign. Through a consistent yoga practice, you eventually discover that there is a mystery beneath the practice that may be heralded in your awareness by the trumpets of a dilemma; however it is all too often exactly at that point—when we run into a paradox—that we pull back from our practice. We divert our attention away from the feelings, thoughts, and sensations that arise in the face of a dilemma, or we seek a different practice in which we will not have to confront the wonder of the paradox. Patterns of avoidance and attachment to certain aspects of the yoga practice naturally arise, and they usually reflect similar patterns that manifest in other facets of our lives; avoidance and attachment to our relationships with other people, to food, our job, money, society, politics, philosophies, and even to our aesthetic tastes. One of the values of a yoga practice is that it teaches us the skill of observing the core patterns of thought, feeling, and sensation that arise within the body as we practice. Gradually this observational skill generalizes into other areas of our life and we become adept at simply observing things as they change. Eventually we can notice core patterns of avoidance and attachment that cause confusion and suffering in all aspects of what we do without reacting to them—without grasping onto them or pushing them away. Slowly the yoga practice exposes root patterns that underlie the complex tapestry of our existence so that the way we approach everything we do and how we relate to the world are influenced by the practice.

Whenever we think about the world or others, we do so via sensations that arise in our own bodies. This is not something that is immediately obvious, but if you go into your thoughts as a meditation it becomes clear. Imagine the core of the body as a set of images for a slide show and that the slides appear not just as images of the way we see things, but that they also manifest in the way we move, talk, and behave. Through the power of our awareness, or consciousness, we project onto the world the slides of our various core patterns of perception. The capacity to discover this principle of projection, which is inherently laced with our tendency to be attracted to or repulsed by different physical feelings, is an invaluable tool for understanding that the world is both given to us and created by us through the way we organize our "slides." For example, if you have watched musicians, you may have noticed that most have unique patterns of holding their body as they go deeply into their music in order to really concentrate on the sound. Some stick their tongue out of their mouth sideways, and others bite their lip, make an odd facial expression, or start tapping their foot wildly. These external physical expressions are fixing a body pattern of sensation to support the focus of the musician's mind. In a less noticeable manner we all do this much of the time: sauntering down the street when we are nervous, speaking loudly when feeling bold, slumping at work when overwhelmed, or gritting our teeth in the face of an argument.

When we practice yoga we cultivate the ability to concentrate the mind so that as we move into various physical postures, we begin to notice our habitual patterns of holding within our own body, just as we might observe physical patterns of holding in musicians as they perform. Say, for example, you are doing a twist in your yoga practice. As you deepen into the pose, your attention drops down and you observe the processes going on within your body and your mind. You may also start to explore different movements you always make and theories you have regarding the composition of the particular pose. You churn these thoughts, feelings, and sensations back and forth as you would blend butter with an old-fashioned hand churn, folding them into the pose and drawing them back out with your mind to mix them back in again. As you work the pose you may start to experience unfamiliar sensations, patterns of deep conditioning that are buried deep within your body. You may have sensations of attachment and also of repulsion to whatever is arising. These habitual patterns and sensations are called saṁskāras. *Sam* means "to collect together" and *kara* refers to activities, deeds, or in this case it refers to things that are made or patterns. Saṁskāras are the subpatterns that are collected together into universal patterns and then held deep inside the body. Our ego structure is intimately tied in to these unconscious configurations, and any good yoga practice takes us right into the heart of our own saṁskāras; it takes us into our deepest pockets of habit. The initial impulse for most of us when faced with our own saṁskāras is to turn away: "Anything but this!" The urge is to run in the opposite direction as fast as possible rather than to deal with habitual ways of perceiving and reacting, because our chronic ways of responding are familiar and comfortable.

In a sense our saṁskāras are quite functional because they allow us to process and react to our perceptions without having to exert the energy and presence of mind required to observe and assess whatever is arising anew. We tend to be creatures of habit, and each of us has unique ways of looking at ourselves and at the world, ways that probably long ago settled within us. These patterns of perception are the result of grasping onto certain things we believe we need or we want, and rejecting other things we believe to be of no use to us or things we imagine are going to hurt us. Deep in the core of the body there is often a kind of anxiety that bubbles up right under the surface of our conscious experience because of our preconceptions about what is good or bad, right or wrong, needed or not needed. The anxiety emerges because a genuine perception of what is actually happening in the present moment is arising, but it is colored by our habitual ways of perceiving—our saṁskāras. Consequently much of our life is spent avoiding the undercurrent of anxiety that surfaces as we place a mask of happiness (or tragedy) over what on a deeper level we are actually aware of—the present moment. With practice we learn to observe these brief little moments of anxiety before they are covered up by the avoidance habits of mind. The content of our observation could be wonderful, bright, and happy, or it could be absolutely miserable, but nonetheless we stick with it and watch it with an open mind and an open heart. And this is the foundation of the practice; that we simply train ourselves to observe the presentation of the mind, the vṛtti, whatever it is and whenever it drifts into our conscious awareness.

Honing this observational skill within āsana, prāṇāyāma, and meditation practice, we eventually discover that there is far more to the practices than we might initially have thought. We find that more important than getting into a remarkably deep back bend, or holding our breath for five minutes, or chanting an entire ancient text from memory, is the power of clear observation. We notice that with practice we become increasingly skilled at noticing the content of our mind before we project its pattern out into our bodies and the world. Most important of all is that we observe our vṛttis as they surface, witnessing what is actually arising through the haze of our saṁskāras of perception. With this type of "in the moment" observation, which is an essential technique in any yoga practice, we slowly begin to break through the most deeply rooted and intimate forms of conditioning that keep us stuck in unhealthy, ineffectual, and unhappy circumstances within our life. The breakthrough happens when we fully comprehend that our conditioned ways of perceiving the world are not only habits of memory, as if we were haunted by dreams, but that they are also physical patterns within the body that over time have rooted themselves in our flesh and in the deepest layers of muscular patterning within our body. When we have a direct experience of this intimate connection between our mind and our physical body, we can then let go and recondition the body, enabling us to be receptive to whatever is arising rather than reacting to it habitually and thereby potentially missing its essence. Clearly observing the vṛtti—the immediate presentation in the mind—as it arises, without accepting or rejecting it, has a profound effect on deep-seated patterns within the body. By shining the light of unobstructed awareness onto whatever we perceive, our saṁskāras gradually become deconditioned and we no longer unconsciously identify whatever feeling we have deep in the core of our being, which habitually has served as the catalyst for that feeling, with the presentation of mind. This process unravels our experience in a way that is exhilarating and joyous, releasing all the accumulated tensions, anxieties, and incomplete experiences that have built up over our lifetime.

The process works because when we observe something we give it space, meaning we temporarily suspend our incessant desire to know it, package it, or compare it to other things. Momentarily, we release whatever it is that we perceive from the label that we automatically—habitually—give it in order to move on quickly and to avoid experiencing it in its full presence. When we give something space we are practicing the physiology of kindness, and we are offering the structure of compassion. This is a gesture of giving respect to whatever the object is and of honoring the environment that the object has come out of. As we pay attention to what is arising in this way, we create what is called tapas or "heat." This is not necessarily a physical heat; it is a metaphorical burning, an awakening to what is really happening within the mind or the perceptions. When people first experience tapas, there is often a sense of discomfort, a desire to squirm away from the situation because it is so authentic; it is as if the border of life is being eaten away by fire. But if we stick with the observational practice, if we do not run away when we reach the juncture where tapas first arises, then we can gain an incredible insight into the fact that all things *do* change. Not only do we understand this conceptually, but we can experience the impression of this principle of transformation within the body; we feel it through our deepest physical sensations, right into the core of the body. When we perceive change in this way and then act with conscious awareness in the face of the present circumstances, we can release our saṁskāras without rejecting them, but instead with an appreciation for their essence. In this way we learn to interact with whatever arises in a more integrated and complete way, whether it is an old pattern of thought or sensation, or a brand-new perception. On the other hand, when our actions are unconscious, when they are driven by our saṁskāras, we end up grasping blindly at things in the world and we act rashly or inappropriately, compounding and magnifying (or avoiding) our problems.

When we practice the yoga of observation and we pay close attention to something, there is a residue of clarity and relief that is discernable in the breath and is actually felt in the body. It is similar to the sensations you might experience when you have been struggling to understand something and then finally "get it," or the feeling you have when you have been deceiving yourself about something and then at last admit to the truth; it is a feeling of relief, openness, cleanliness, and joy. We experience this when we pay close attention to things as they arise because we are directly perceiving, rather than distorting our observation by imagining that things are the way we expect or want them to be. Simple, clear observation allows us to cut through our own layers of programming, preconception, and habitual perception. When our saṁskāras are suspended, instead of experiencing a sense of anxiety due to tension between our projections and the truth, we may experience a deep sense of physical relief within the body; the glorious feeling of the residue of truth. It is really quite straightforward. As we continue to practice yoga we find that sometimes we are able to observe closely without much influence from our habitual patterns, and we also become aware of those times when we are driven completely by our old habits of mind and body. Gradually we train both body and mind to be awake, and, little by little, we decondition ourselves from the habits that keep us dull and stuck in the routine of our own suffering. We cultivate

Temple of Awareness

the ability to observe clearly rather than using an iron hand to squelch the urges driven by our saṁskāras. Having habitual responses to things as they arise is a perfectly natural state of affairs, so the practice and the work become to watch these patterns as they arise and to foster within ourselves the ability to not react, project, or overlay our preconceptions. Our very own body, which is immediately available to us, becomes a laboratory of consciousness, a field of exploration into the truth of our own existence so that, figuratively speaking, our body becomes a temple for open awareness.

3

The Process of Haṭha Yoga
Union of Sun and Moon

suṣmnāyai kuṇḍalinyai sudhāyai
candrajanmane
manonmanyai namastubhyaṁ mahāśaktyai
cidātmane

Salutations to the Suṣumnā, to the Kuṇḍalinī,
and to the nectar originating from the moon.
Salutations to you, the Unmani mind,
to the great śakti, to pure Being as contentless awareness.

—*Haṭha Yoga Pradīpikā,* IV. 64

The epigraph at the beginning of this chapter is a series of salutations, first to the suṣumnā nāḍī, which is the channel that lies along the central axis of the body and is considered itself to be the guru. The verse then offers salutations to the kuṇḍalinī, the sleeping, coiled energy of pure consciousness that when awakened moves through this central channel. Next salutations are offered to sudhā, or the nectar, that flows from the moon at the bottom of the sahasrāra or the thousand-petalled lotus cakra at the crown of the head. The chant offers salutations to the one who erases the mind, facilitating liberation from mental constructs, and finally salutations are given to the mahāśakti, the great power that is the universe and the one who is the pure intelligence of the self, or pure being. The contemplation of the awakening of the suṣumnā nāḍī in this way is the entire purpose of the practice of haṭha yoga.

When we practice yoga we wake up the body. We concentrate the mind on different fields of sensation, which awakens the core of the body and, in turn, allows us to experience deep feelings. This is the body-mind connection. Whenever we think about something on a profound level, we create a physical pattern or a combination of sensations within the body that allows us to hold the thought. Through this process we associate certain things in the outside world with specific sensations and core feelings within the depths of our body. It is a somewhat arbitrary process in which we happen to have connected together the two in our subconscious mind, and the association sticks. It is kind of like a Pavlovian response—when after years away from home, we walk into our mother's kitchen and begin to drool. It can happen that gradually the body becomes dull and desensitized because old abstractions and concepts, past desires and fears, or previous experiences have settled into patterns of feeling in our body. We start to believe these patterns to be real rather than recognizing them as associations with earlier experiences or thoughts. When this happens, these stagnant patterns continue to generate stuck thoughts and fixed reactions. We become restricted in our thinking and so contracted in our perception of immediate feelings and sensations that our bodies become shriveled-up forms, not manifesting their true liberated potential.

Grounded in physical practices, the haṭha yoga system examines the body with a fine-tooth comb—pulling open different internal sensations and feelings, waking up whole fields and entire spectrums of sensation and feeling that may have been lying dormant for years deep within the body. Gradually we are able to separate our saṁskāras (patterns of stagnant feelings and sensations that are associated with the past) from the feelings and sensations that are in response to input we are receiving right here, right now. We learn to differentiate in this way from the tips of our toes, to our fingers, right up our spinal column, and through the crown of the head. We find that when we practice yoga all of these fields of sensitivity—which penetrate the entire body like the tiny filaments inside of a flower—are awakened; every thought, every movement of the mind travels through these fibers of sensitivity in the core of the body.

The way we hold and move our bodies reflects a history of perception patterns, thoughts about the world, mental maps charting territory inside and outside the body, as well as movement patterns and the reactions we received from them. The flesh has embodied our mental and emotional history, and as long as it is alive it provides lessons and even opportunities to find freedom and understanding from mental confusion. Yoga āsana practice when done mindfully is a minitheater of the mind and heart, teaching both visceral and intellectual truths to the attentive. For example, a beginner first practices the triangle pose by following simple instructions; that is, "Open the legs about one leg length apart. Turn the right foot out and line it up with the front edge of the heel of the back foot. Inhaling, lift the arms, and then exhaling, reach out through the right arm and rotate the pelvis around so that you can place your hand on the floor near the right ankle, or hold the right big toe with the middle and index fingers." These verbal instructions, though accurate, would function better with a personal demonstration or at least a drawing or some sort of illustration. The difficulty is obvious: even with personal instruction the technique is complicated to transmit, and even more challenging to convey is how the intelligence must work with technique in order to make the āsana a transparent fountain of meditation and insight.

Every turn, every spiral, every extension eventually has to be tempered by a counterturn, a counterspiral, or a flexion; sometimes strong, sometimes subtle. Each instruction or technique, at the right time, will need a counterinstruction or technique to find openness and balance. Mindful observation, to the extent that samādhi may spontaneously arise, is gradually cultivated in āsana. We practice so that on a mental level, our theories about the techniques, our sectarian and political attachments to them, and even our need to prove a theistic or metaphysical theory, can be observed impartially and recognized as context dependent. The fine-tooth comb of āsana practice will bring up the knots and tangles of past and present misperceptions and their embodiment in deep holding patterns in the body. What we call alignment is a continuous balancing

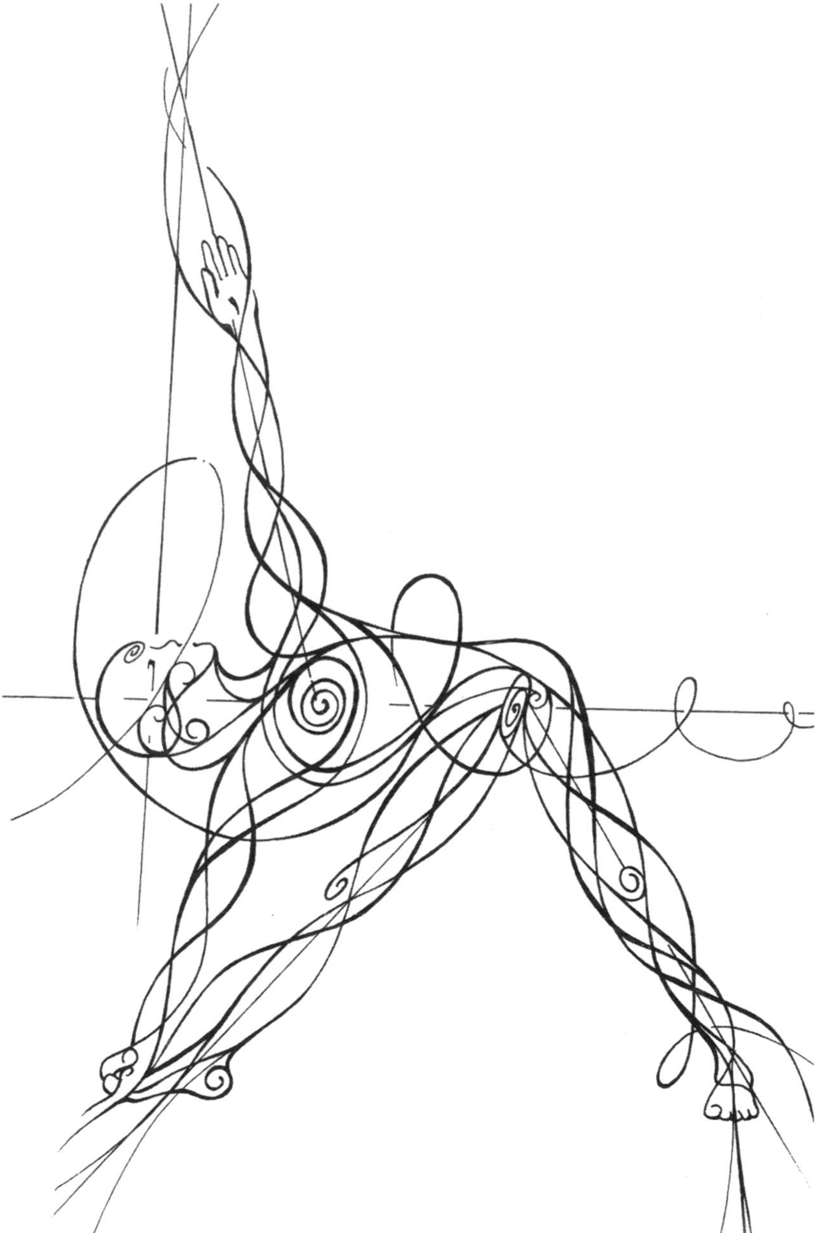

and interpenetrating of opposites on many levels, starting from muscular movement patterns within the complete wave of a full breath and moving on through the ever more subtle layers of body and mind. Alignment is a steady flame of intelligence.

Through a well-aligned āsana practice we begin to recognize that feelings and sensations are integrally connected to the breath. It is said that the mind and the inner breath move together like two fish swimming in tandem; when the mind moves in a particular pattern, the fish of the inner breath moves along with it through the core of the body, hitting deep sensations and feelings as it moves. Likewise, if that inner fish of the breath moves in a certain way, it stimulates or wakes up associated patterns of thought or imagination within the mind. The connection between these two fish forms a basic axiom that we use for yoga practice: the joining of opposites. One fish is called prāṇa, the inner breath. Prāṇa is the way we pattern sensations and feelings into recognizable forms. The other fish is called citta, or the mind. It is said that when either prāṇa or citta vibrates, the other does so equally. If we are able to become aware of the vibrations of either prāṇa or citta, or better yet if we can control one of them, then we have a handle on the other one. This relation between the mind and the breath is the most elemental

The Triangle Pose (2)

The triangle pose, trikoṇāsana, has many opposing structural movements and forces that come together to wake up a toned intelligence in the pelvic floor, the center of which is represented as a triangle in the tantric tradition. The internally rotating spiraling patterns radiate outward and are involved with prāṇa, which controls the inhaling breath. The externally rotating spiraling patterns contract back in toward the core and are associated with the apāna, which controls the exhaling breath. The prāṇa and the apāna are balanced, interfaced, and squeezed together to form the internal, meditative movement of the posture. The eyes become steady in soft gazing (dṛṣṭi) and the ears open to give space to all of the elements of the body. When the alignment of the posture is well tuned, it is easy to trace the central axis of the body on through the crown of the head, and the posture and its residue are conducive to deep meditation.

trick, the "secret," of the deep, bodily oriented practice called haṭha yoga because by shaping and stretching and thereby freeing the breath we can liberate the mind. Through haṭha yoga practices we can actually begin to identify the physiological processes that are at the root of our mind. Of course it is the mind that causes suffering, but the very same mind allows for liberation and freedom. By unlinking the physical patterns of breath that lie within our body from the antics of our mind, we can allow both body and mind to work more intelligently, and eventually, rather than perpetuating our own suffering, we can begin to make inroads into our release from suffering.

The inner breath, the prāṇa, is considered to be the substratum of all sensation, feeling, and thought, the medium through which all experience within the body presents itself. There are many subdivisions of prāṇa that describe the wide range of its movements and patterns inside the body, but two are most important for our yoga practice: prāṇa and apāna. Prāṇa is the physical pattern of rising up, blossoming, and spreading out. Prāṇa's direct opposite is the pattern of apāna, a downward, contracting, rooting movement. (Note that the word *prāṇa* is used to describe both the pattern of the inhaling breath as well as the general idea of inner breath, which can sometimes cause confusion.) If you imagine a tree, you can envision a similar system, with a joining of an expansive pattern (associated with prāṇa) and a grounding pattern (associated with apāna). The roots that reach down into the earth find the nutrients necessary for the growth and survival of the tree. Because of this rooting, this nourishment from the earth, the top of the tree has the capacity for expansion as the leaves and flowers of the tree are exposed to air, sunlight, and open sky. Without the stability and nutrients that the roots provide, the expansion at the top of the tree is not possible, and without the expression of life in the upper part of the tree, there is no point to the rooting; with no inspiration to grow, the desire to push through the soil and root is not stimulated. The two patterns need each other intimately. It is said that in the heart of prāṇa is apāna, and in the heart of apāna is prāṇa. They are like two lovers—yin and yang in the Chinese Taoist system—each in the heart of the other. Actually, they are inseparable. Similarly, we may separate the concepts of prāṇa and apāna in our mind in order to be able to think about them, to talk about them, and to experience them, but just as the roots and the top of a tree are divided only in order for our minds to be able to comprehend the different functions they serve, so too the prāṇa and the apāna are never truly separate.

The apāna is believed to reside in the mūlādhāra cakra, which is located at the perineum, and it is said to wind itself up into a coil to be stored like a kernel or a seed at this central point of the pelvic floor. The prāṇa is thought to dwell at the core of the heart, or the anāhata cakra. It is possible to determine the character of the two aspects of breath and to feel their resting points within your own body by tracing the flow of your breath. The expansive, upward rising and spreading pattern of prāṇa, is experienced physically when we inhale. If you simply observe internally and watch the flow of the prāṇa as you take a full, slow, conscious in-breath, you will notice that the pattern begins down around the navel. Continuing the inhalation, there is a sense of rising and spreading that becomes full and wide as the expansion of the breath moves along the edges of the diaphragm. This spacious pattern increases, spreading and blossoming as it rises into the heart area, where it often stimulates the mind, causing us to wander off into the realm of thinking. There is a moment when the tree of the breath comes to full bloom at the top of the inhale, and then all of a sudden everything changes and the apanic pattern takes over. There is a gradual releasing of the breath, and the expansive sensations associated with prāṇa are replaced by feelings of drawing in to the core of the body, dropping, stability, and of being grounded as the exhale squeezes down and roots into the base of the pelvic floor, tethering body and mind to the earth. One helpful method of understanding the relationship between prāṇa and apāna is to think about the seasons. The beginning of the in-breath is like the start of spring, filled with the potential for new life and with plants budding and flowering trees filled with delicate leaves. As the blossoms or trees come to full bloom they are surrounded by excited bumblebees, and there is a great sense of optimism and potential for life. Then the season begins to shift: summer arrives and passes. As the fruit ripens and fall approaches, sap in the tree begins to come back into the trunk, and plants secure themselves into the earth, signaling the transition to a time when dropping roots deep down is of paramount importance. Leaves and flowers begin to fall off until by the dead of winter there are no leaves left, and all of the life force is buried deep in the ground. After some time, with the first signs of spring, bulbs break through frozen ground, the trees begin to wake up, and the first signs of sprouts appear at the end of the branches. This cyclical pattern of expansion into full bloom, followed by a rooting into the ground of what could be considered our awareness, is characteristic of the relation of the prāṇa and the apāna within our own bodies.

The underlying process of haṭha yoga is to explore deeply this relationship of the inhale and the exhale; to discover the root of apāna in the prāṇa, and the expansion of prāṇa in the apāna. We do this initially by observing and cultivating opposite physiological patterns within the body. When we inhale and the expansive, blossoming pattern naturally manifests, we allow the awareness of mind to drop down to the root of the body and the breath, to the perineum, and beyond that to the legs and feet, which are extensions of the pelvic floor keeping us connected to the earth. Rather than becoming distracted by one of the metaphorical branches of the "tree" that is manifesting through the inhaling breath, we focus on the roots of the breath. Then as we exhale, when the pranic rooting pattern is naturally dominant and we may tend to become distracted by the serious quality of the exhale, we allow our mind to remain in the center of the heart so that we relish and maintain awareness of the essence of the flowering pranic pattern that is still within the body, until we reach the end of the exhale and begin the inhaling pattern anew. When we do not consciously experience the unity of the inhale and exhale we lose touch with the essential qualities of the pattern of each: as we exhale, we ignore the basic qualities of the inhaling pattern, and conversely as we inhale we lose touch with the characteristics of the exhaling pattern. The result is that at some point during the out-breath we close our heart, or during the in-breath wc become overwhelmed by its expansive feeling so that we become completely ungrounded. This happens as a result of an attachment to or a repulsion for something we associate with one of the inherent patterns of the breath: a saṁskāra that is stirred by the feelings of either the flowering or the rooting pattern of breath. For this reason it is perfectly normal that as we exhale, a feeling of anxiety—an overwhelming sense that is akin to the fear of death—arises because the apanic pattern stimulates physical sensations associated with change and dissolution. At some point during the exhale it is quite common that the heart closes and all the physiological patterns of prāṇa within the body disappear. Conversely, when we inhale, at some point as the rising and spreading pattern extends out through the body, we may become overwhelmed by an aspect of the expansion so that we lose connection to our roots and the pranic pattern, and we float away. We become lost in our imagination because it is so stimulating at the top of the inhale. In yoga practice, whenever we are inhaling, we remain focused on staying grounded so as not to project a sense of essence and "thingness" out into the tips of the sensation tree of prāṇa. When we exhale we realize that the essence is in the core of the heart, so we allow the leaves and flowers of the tree of our breath to fall away without experiencing anxiety or fear in response to the apānic pattern of dissolution. Of course this is very simply said and much more difficult to actually do, but it sums up the essence of what we are cultivating within the study of haṭha yoga even as we practice the āsana.

The uniting of the ends of the breath is also the underlying process of a prāṇāyāma practice, which, along with āsana, is a foundational form of practice within haṭha yoga. Prāṇāyāma could be explained as various techniques for breathing that consciously join prāṇa and apāna as a means of freeing the inner breath so that it can unfold into its true liberated state. Bringing awareness to the breath through a prāṇāyāma practice, consciously working to maintain awareness within the transitions of the inhale and the exhale, and learning to stretch the breath, is essential within the haṭha yoga tradition. It is said that the severing of prāṇa and apāna is the experience of death and that yoga is the opposite of death; it is the conscious joining of prāṇa and apāna. With a great deal of practice, in particular while doing the yoga postures, we learn to observe the in-breath as an integral part of the out-breath, and the exhale as inherent to the inhale, so that through consistent practice we eventually experience physically how the intertwining and the interplay of these two breathing patterns affect the entire structure of the body and the mind.

Eventually we are able to take the essence of the apānic pattern, that of grounding, and draw it up along the central axis of the body into the roots of our navel. At the same time we are able to connect with the prāṇic pattern, the flowering centered at the core of the heart, and we can press that pattern down into the roots of the navel. We learn to consciously join prāṇa and apāna where they meet, causing an ignition of awareness in the plane of the navel, which then creates an experience of intense inner heat and ecstasy. Some consider this to be the primary initiation into the inner world of yoga practice. This is why the patron saint of haṭha yoga, Gaṇeśa, the elephant-headed god who symbolizes the awakened kuṇḍalinī, has a big belly. In fact, as can be seen in illustrations of Gaṇeśa, his entire body represents the processes of haṭha yoga. He has a huge belly, and wrapped around his navel is a cobra, and right at that navel point the heads of the multiheaded cobra are opening and lifting, symbolizing the joining of prāṇa with apāna. Gaṇeśa's lower belly is scooped out, way down underneath the cobra, in order to pull the apāna up into the roots of the navel, and his belly has expanded so much that it is as if a flower—the pranic pattern—had initiated its bloom at the base of his navel as well. Gaṇeśa's hips are extremely open, and he is extraordinarily grounded and solid, indicating that the rooting apānic pattern is well established. His elephant head has an exceptionally long nose—for the practice of prāṇāyāma—and his large ears facilitate listening so that he can hear pure sound in the deepest meditation, the most profound samādhi. Gaṇeśa is also known to have a fantastic sense of humor and is considered to be the intelligence itself. His extreme bodily form is a lesson in not taking the metaphors that describe the yogic process too literally. After all, who really has an elephant head? So Gaṇeśa is laughing with us at the silliness of our own minds: that we grasp onto images and onto myths, that we hold on to as idols our very means of understanding. He laughs along with us that we take these symbols literally when their metaphorical value is so much more profound and rich than their literal representations could ever be.

When we open and unfold both body and mind through haṭha yoga we connect with our "yogic body," which can take on many forms and which is actually quite imaginary. In fact, contemplating imagery within the body or even *thinking* about what a subtle state of body *might* feel like is a great way to begin working into the more subtle, internal aspects of yoga. For instance, you can imagine channels of breath like bright tubes opening up from one central channel into branches that then return into a single central tube within the core of your body. This is a common image, taught to help practitioners connect with the flow of the inner breath. In haṭha yoga these imagined tubes are usually referred to as nāḍīs. *Nāḍī* means "little river." For most of us, our small rivers of breath and energy are all clogged up. Some of the rivers flow just a little bit, others not at all, and some are flooding our system the entire time. In other words, the subtle flow of the breath throughout the body is not balanced. The nāḍīs become blocked by our saṁskāras, our old abstractions, thoughts, feelings, and desires. The physical patterning associated with these experiences—our habits of observation, the tapes that keep playing themselves over and over again within our mind—cause imbalanced flow and obstructions within the nāḍīs. These blockages are patterns of separation and of fear that serve to deaden the connection between the body and mind, and which cause the mind to become dull. This is a root cause of suffering. The goal of the process of haṭha yoga is simply to clean out whatever is impinging the currents of movement within the nāḍīs so that we can get an even and complete flow of breath and energy throughout the entire body, thus automatically awakening the natural intelligence that lies within.

Different classical yogic texts refer to different numbers of nāḍīs; some say 72,000, others 100,000, and some even 300,000. It does not really matter how many there are (or whether, in fact, they are real or imagined), the point is that there are innumerable small rivers of breath throughout the body. All texts that mention nāḍīs give special importance to three of them in the practice of yoga: the iḍā, the piṅgalā and the suṣumnā nāḍīs. The iḍā is considered to be the moon channel, which is said to be cooling and calming and is accessible through the sensations in your left nostril. The piṅgalā, which is accessed through feelings in your right nostril, is considered to be the sun channel and is thought to be heating and energizing. From a yogic perspective, these two channels of the prāṇa are also associated with different states of mind, with the iḍā considered to be feminine, and the piṅgalā masculine. It is said that when you stimulate one of these two primary nāḍīs you experience characteristic moods and modes of thinking associated with the temperament of that side. The suṣumnā nāḍī is the empty channel, the hollow reed, right in the core of the body, and it can be accessed through what is called the "root of the palate." Physiologically, the root of the palate begins in the soft palate located in the back of the roof of the mouth where the uvula hangs down. The root is like a cup immediately under the pituitary gland. To access the root of your palate you must first tune into and become aware of the roof of your mouth. If you could slide the tip of the tongue up along the back edge of the nasal septum, you would come to the area of this "root." Sometimes, if you eat really fine food and fully experience the merging of flavor and aroma within the mouth, you automatically connect to the root of the palate. The connection also happens naturally when you have an experience of profound beauty, which can automatically connect you to the seed of aestheticism deep within, reflexively awakening the root of the palate. The link to this seed point within the body causes you to spontaneously smile in a very soft and subtle way—like the *Mona*

KUNDALINI-CHAKRA (3) power of universal intellegence

When the practice of prāṇāyāma cleans the nāḍīs and allows the mind to concentrate easily in meditation, the apāna can drop strongly and evenly through the four corners of the pelvic floor. This balances and then suspends the flow of the inner breath through the iḍā and the piṅgalā. The pressing together of prāṇa and apāna in the navel chakra (nabhi chakra) creates a type of inner heat that causes the kuṇḍalinī to uncoil from her grip, which blocks the entrance to the suṣumnā nāḍī. When prāṇa begins to flow in this central channel it balances and opens, from both below and above, all of the chakras that are strung like flowers on a thread. The spreading cobra hoods over the crown of the head represent the complete unfolding of the great power of the universal intelligence that holds the mind suspended effortlessly in its natural state of pure awareness.

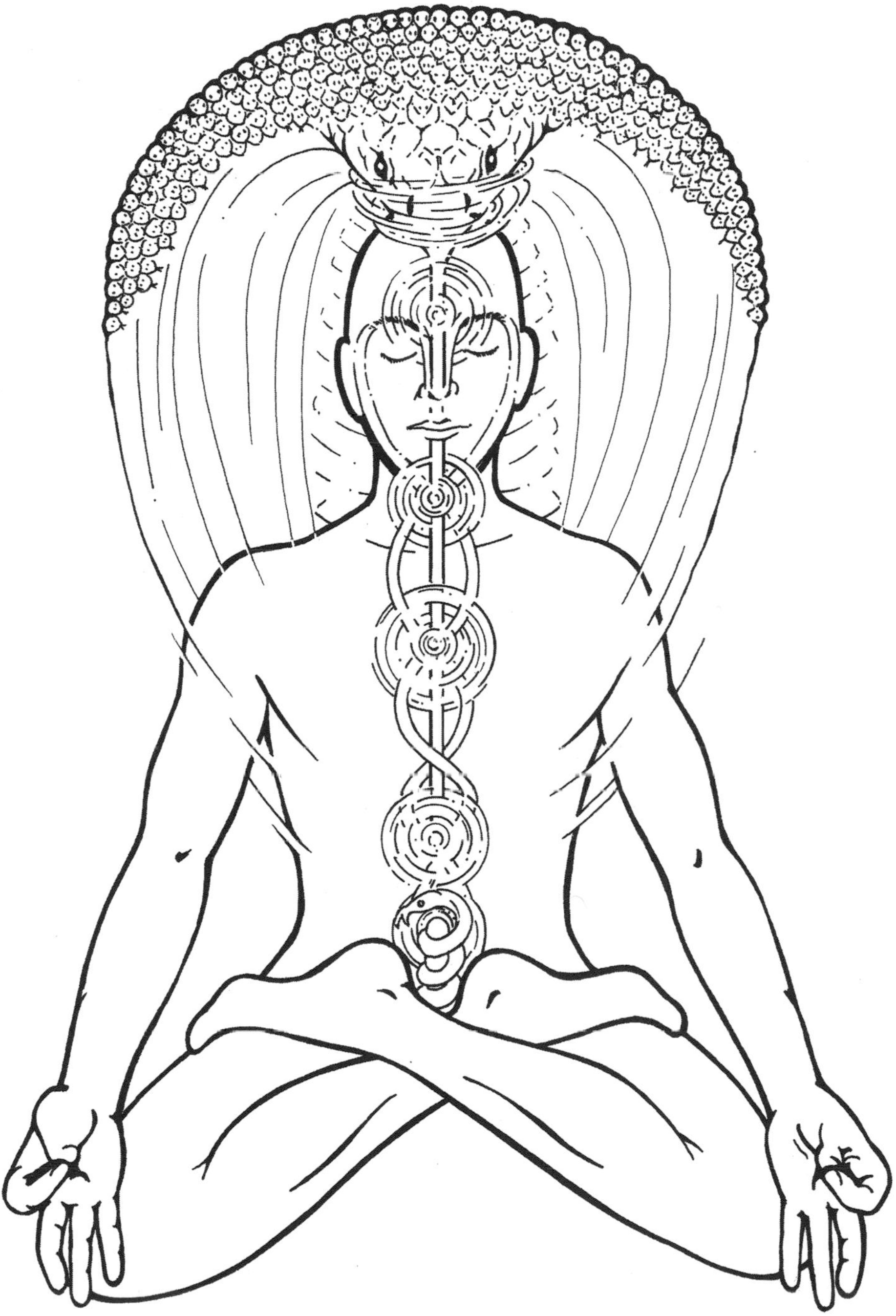

Lisa. Yogic texts describe a beautiful, bright, endlessly extending flower called the sahasrāra, or the "thousand-petaled lotus," originating at the roor of the palate and opening through and beyond the crown of the head. From the soft palate, back and up into the base of the sahasrāra is the gateway into the central channel. Here the three nāḍīs, the central staff of the suṣumnā, the iḍā (the moon channel), and the piṅgalā (the sun channel), form an image that is somewhat like the caduceus, the wand of Hermes in Greek mythology, which is entwined by serpents. Just as the snakes wrap around the caduceus of life and work their way around the staff in subtle, smooth motion, so too the opposing qualities of the breath and subtle body intertwine and have their resolution in the central axis.

This kind of internal imagery encourages us to observe both subtle and more blatant effects of the breath. In addition to affecting the way you feel physically, the flow of the prāṇa makes a difference in how you map out an awareness of the core of the body, and it influences the type of thinking you do—more practical or more abstract—as it impacts different tendencies of mind. It is said that when the left nostril is more open and the moon channel is stimulated, you become more receptive; you might be more melancholy and are likely to have thoughts that are pluralistic in nature. You might have more of an appreciation for the fact that in the night sky there are millions and billions of suns or stars. Conversely, when the sun channel is stimulated through the right nostril, it is believed that you become more active and that your perspective will likely be dominated by perceptions of the one rather than the many. In this case you are more likely to engage in the world around you, making plans with decisive confidence. Of course, with close observation you will notice that just as you think you have understood the underlying pattern of your breath and how it is affecting you, the dominant nostril shifts sides, and the quality of the breath, and all of your theories about it, change. It is just like when the sun rises at dawn: we forget about the beauty and wonder of the nighttime stars, we grab a cup of coffee, and make a list. Depending on which channel of breath is more dominant, you either become too externally oriented or too internally focused. A true yoga practice occurs when you get the two channels of prāṇa balanced, leading to a spontaneous sense of harmony between inner and outer focus and states of mind. The foundation of a haṭha yoga practice becomes the act of observing your breath flow shifting and balancing so that you can track its effect on changes in the patterns of your awareness and in how you imagine yourself and your world. Notice any sunlike temptation to reduce your observations to just a theory. Instead, stay with the open, vibrating quality of the breath and everything within it.

Many of explanations of the qualities of breath and the nāḍīs found in Indian texts are filled with rich imagery similar to that found in Greek mythology, for example, the caduceus. If you contemplate these images, you might find that they stimulate within you feelings associated with energy flow through the nāḍīs that the images represent. Of course it might not happen (especially if you really want it to), but you can always experiment to see if there is any truth to the idea of an image stimulating physical feelings. As human beings we sometimes become so excited about our theories, our blueprints, or conceptual systems that we superimpose our concepts onto the real data with which we are presented. You should never take anyone's word for theories like this—that the channels of breath represent the sun and the moon, or that they are either masculine or feminine, or even that there *are* channels of breath within the body. Instead, consider these constructs and ideas as an invitation to explore for yourself. If you observe the flow of the breath in your own nostrils, you will probably notice that it shifts from side to side over the course of the day. In fact, it is quite common that every hour and a half the flow of the breath shifts from being dominant on one side to being dominant on the other. You may find that the side that is more open is more stimulated, and also that there is more sensation in the nostril and sinus passages on that side of the body. On occasion you may observe the two sides merging or dissolving into the central channel. Your own body is a convenient and rich resource for experimentation and for understanding the principles and theories presented in haṭha and tantric yoga texts.

It is interesting to note that the *Haṭha Yoga Pradīpikā*, an important medieval yogic text, presents the idea that one should not practice

Svāra

meditation with focus on the core of the body during the day or during the night. This makes it sound as though you are off the hook and that you do not really need to meditate at all, but that is not the meaning of the statement. Rather it is code language for the idea that you cannot truly meditate on the core of the body if the iḍā and the piṅgalā are out of balance. Through the focused and consistent practice of yoga āsana and prāṇāyāma, the iḍā and the piṅgalā automatically become balanced, which allows for the potential of the opening of the suṣumnā nāḍī and a full connection to a profound and deep meditative state of mind. Hence, the word *haṭha* (*ha* meaning "sun," *ṭha* meaning "moon") refers to the sun channel and the moon channel becoming balanced or conjoined so that the central channel is opened for meditation practice. The relationship between the sun and the moon channels, like the relationship between day and night or the left and the right wings of a bird, is endlessly fascinating. There are entire systems of divination and ancient medicine based on the theory of the joining of opposite patterns, such as the flow of breath in the channels of the body. Many of these systems of thought include the belief that it is good luck to carry out certain activities when one of the two opposing patterns—perhaps the sun or moon channel—is dominant. All of this could be considered to be old wives' tales or folk medicine, but who knows? How feelings, sensations, thoughts, and activities change when the breath flow in the nostrils is dominant on one side or the other is, at the very least, an interesting idea and something to experiment with, to observe within your own practice.

One common yogic practice is to purposely switch the dominance of one side of the breath over to the other side. It is very easy to do; you simply lie down on the side that has the more dominant flow of breath, and use the upper arm on that side as you would a pillow for resting your head. The restriction of the circulation in the shoulder area on the side you are lying on reflexively causes the sinuses on the opposite side to open so that the flow of breath, the svāra, switches sides in dominance. This reflex is built into the body; it is quite fascinating. Even if you have a deviated septum, the air flow shifts dominance over the course of the day and during this simple exercise. With a deviated septum the physical sensations are more subtle, so you must be more observant of obscure shifts in the breath, but you can still control the flow of the breath and track the svāra. Another traditional practice that is used for bringing a sense of balance into the body is to consciously switch the flow of the svāra from side to side several times in a row, in order to bring it back into a point of balance. We find that when we do yoga āsana and prāṇāyāma this balance naturally occurs, and at the end of a good practice there is a sense of internal balance, as if the breath is flowing evenly between the iḍā and piṅgalā or possibly that it is resting in the suṣumnā nāḍī. If you practice yoga regularly and this level of balance does not come quickly, it could be an indication that you are getting ill, but it is more likely a sign that you are not practicing with internal form and awareness. Again, as with all of the practices, these are simply indicators to be observed, reference points for awareness, as you cultivate a sense of deepening the practice.

When you do find balance of the breath, if you have even a glimpse of uniting the complementary principles of the sun and the moon channels, something very interesting begins to occur at the mūlādhāra cakra, which holds the root of the breath channels in the pelvic floor. According to yogic theory, the two streams of breath are allowed to unite when we remove the blockage that is between them. This obstruction is called the kuṇḍalinī. The root of the word, *kuṇḍa,* means a "coil," leading to the word *kuṇḍalinī* and conjuring the image of a coiled serpent lying asleep right at the base of the breath in the pelvic floor, in the very spot where the prāṇa and apāna are attempting to unite. This "coiled serpent" (or the energetic feeling that this serpent represents) interferes with the interpenetrating relationship of the sun and the moon channels, and it also inhibits their ability to enter into the suṣumnā nāḍī. The skillful practice of haṭha yoga removes this blockage, allowing the two aspects of the breath to unite and flow easily and unobstructed into the central channel so that deep levels of meditation or samādhi can spontaneously arise. This arising is considered to be the freeing of the prāṇa, which can then be referred to as the Prāṇa Devatā, the goddess Prāṇa, liberated to flow evenly in the central channel. Indeed, under these circumstances the breath is free because it is no longer restricted

yama. constrict, control
a yāma. to set loose

by our preconceptions and our desires and the entire complex of core and habitual feelings, thoughts, and sensations we hold in the body. When the prāṇa finds its way to the central channel and is set free in this way, it radiates out through the rest of the body, just like the sun, casting out light and releasing radiance continuously. It is also believed that at this time, the vibration of the prāṇa in the nāḍīs that are peripheral to the central axis ceases. In other words, the breath becomes still and concentrated in the central channel, allowing the mind to settle so that the patterns of the agitation of feelings, thoughts, and sensations that are associated with the prāṇa moving through the rest of the body (the peripheral nāḍīs) also settle. As a result, the normal world-constructing, world-interpreting activities of the mind are temporarily suspended, and the mind enters into a state of awe and pure attention, which is focused along the central axis of our being. At this point, it is believed that the internal breath, the kuṇḍalinī, uncoils and stands up straight along the central axis—just as a coiled snake lifts up straight out of its coiled state when alert.

This spiraling and uncoiling action of the breath is truly the meaning of prāṇāyāma, which is a joining of the two words, *prāṇa* and *ayāma*. *Yāma* means "to constrict, to control," so *ayāma,* the opposite, means "to set loose," "to free or extend," "to expand or unfold." Prāṇāyāma is the practice of breathing exercises in which we extend the length and the smoothness of inhaling and of exhaling to discover any difficulties in the patterns of the prāṇa and the apāna. After some practice, prāṇāyāma becomes a deliberate suspension of the breath that allows the mind to become extremely focused and calm, since it is the movement of the breath that actually makes the mind move. Gradually through our prāṇāyāma practice the suspension or retention of the breath becomes easy and spontaneous and starts to have a deep effect in the core of the body. An immediate result is that the nāḍīs become purified, and the inner ear opens so we are able to listen very, very deeply. In that listening we learn to give space to all of the other elements of the mind and body so that we can observe them without bias. This is how prāṇāyāma works; it releases the bonds that restrict the prāṇa, setting the breath free. The feelings and sensations associated with the awakening of the breath are sometimes compared to a very thin, beautiful chain of lightening. There are many metaphors describing the delicacy, precision, and beauty associated with the releasing of the bonds of the breath, the awakened suṣumnā and the movement of kuṇḍalinī along the central channel. Some practitioners visualize different forms of their preferred goddess or god standing up through their entire body, making every sensation or extension of their mind an aspect of the divine body, down to the most precise and intricate detail.

Because these images of uncoiled snakes and vibrating gods or goddesses standing upright at the base of the pelvis are so vivid and colorful, the idea of the kuṇḍalinī awakening is universally appealing. It is also very easy for the mind to understand the images and to hold on to the ideas they represent. In fact, the kuṇḍalinī rising is such an attractive image that we may hold too tightly to our vision of it, and in so doing avoid the actual experience if we happen to encounter it. It is important to remember that the process of yoga is really the observation of what *is*, not the reduction of what is to our theory about it, or to our images of what we would like it to be. Kuṇḍalinī is a metaphorical description of what could be a direct experience of reality in the present moment, but if our image of the snake awakening along our central channel is so wildly appealing that we grasp it, hang our imagination on to it, put it up on a pedestal, then we short circuit any chance we might have of actually experiencing the prāṇa entering the central channel. When we practice yoga we get tastes of this—both the grasping and the release—just as we encounter snippets of the actual experiences that yoga can stimulate. In fact, the mystical experience is something that many, many people have, whether or not they do yoga. But if they have no context in which to explain their experience, either they forget about it or they try to fit it into their favorite imagery, beloved religion, or interpretive system, rather than simply observing the whole experience as it is. The joining of prāṇa with apāna, the appearance of kuṇḍalinī, or the spontaneous arising of a mystical experience are all aspects of existence that yoga can contextualize and ground in the actual experience of everyday, ordinary existence so that we can become more present, more authentic, and more compassionate.

Within the haṭha yoga tradition, the awakening of the central axis is, by definition, the end of the manifestation of time and space. It is actually the process of finding the deepest, true root of the mind. At times, this spontaneously happens during a yoga practice; the normal external conceptualization process of the mind instinctively stops, at which point the yoga actually begins to work. So the kuṇḍalinī, even the yoga practice itself, may not be what you think it is. This is because the mind likes to take its experiences and hand them over to the ego, which then wants to package everything for its own purposes. This is very normal; everyone does it. If we have had a mystical experience we may associate and confuse the things that were the content of the mind at the time we had the mystical experience with the experience itself. This is the natural degeneration of an ecstatic state of mind into a dull state of mind, and it happens all the time. When we are first practicing yoga we may get little shots of current through the central channel, little "ahhhhs!" little feelings of inspiration. But because the entire system of the nāḍīs is not yet cleared and cleaned through the practice of āsana and prāṇāyāma, our experience of the movement of the breath and energy in the central channel is fleeting. Nonetheless, the mind quickly interprets our experience and tries to bring it back into the ego structure in order to make sense of it, as a means of giving it a context. Consequently, many people will believe (or claim with glee) that their kuṇḍalinī has awakened because they have had a taste of it, or because they believe the imagery to be true and they consider the idea of an awakened kuṇḍalinī to be fashionable, not because they have actually had an integrated mystical experience. Sometimes if this happens to us as yoga students, our yoga teacher, out of a sense of kindness, may encourage us and say, oh yes, that is kuṇḍalinī awakening, when in fact every sensation and every feeling in the entire universe is kuṇḍalinī. The symptom of a true awakening is that one has the astonishing realization that the entire universe is merely the vibration we call prāṇa, and that *all* of our experience is in its essence empty of any permanent form and is empty of separateness from everything else.

Some say that when the kuṇḍalinī awakens the entire universe disappears, which sounds like a good indicator for recognizing a true awakening of kuṇḍalinī. Perhaps a more practical and significant way to understand the kuṇḍalinī is to remember that all haṭha yoga practices are extremely real and grounded, so that if a yoga practice does not encourage a sense of grounding, then it is not being practiced correctly and an actual awakening of the kuṇḍalinī is not possible. When you practice non-exotic, everyday yoga—looking deeply at the ordinary experience, becoming more honest and more kind—there is a great sense of relief. You are freed from fantasy, freed even from contrived associations with the image of kuṇḍalinī as a snake arising within you, and freed from ego-centered notions of the cakras. This approach to yoga is grounded in an understanding and experience of impermanence. It invites you to come into the present moment and intuitively know what is truly essential, so that you connect instinctively into a state that is called jñāna, or "wisdom." You experience a sense of discriminative insight in which you do not confuse the word that represents something, or the image of that thing, with the actual thing itself. For example, you experience someone you love—your spouse, your child, or your dog—as a deep and wondrous being, but you do not project onto them your habitual labels, your needs or desires. Essentially, when you experience discriminative insight, you do not pull anything out of its background. Instead you see everything, including a being you love, just as it is, and your perceptions are not clouded by an overlay of theories, preconceptions, and expectations. Discriminative awareness is a form of intelligence that can be experienced as a sense of razor sharpness of the mind on all levels of consciousness and knowledge. When you experience this form of wisdom known as jñāna, it is accompanied by what is called vairāgyam, or complete nonattachment. This is because when things are seen as interpenetrating manifestations of the whole, you are quite naturally filled with a sense of respect and awe for all different levels of manifestation. This is true whether what you perceive is experienced deep inside your own heart or as not part of you at all. So discriminative awareness and complete nonattachment are the two symptoms of actual awakening that occur spontaneously through a steady and internal yoga practice. If both of these states do not manifest naturally as you practice, then you are having what would be considered a distorted reflection of the yogic processes. It can still be a magnificent experience, but it is not the complete yogic experience and it is not the actual awakening of kuṇḍalinī, the dissolving of the entire world in the vision of empty, open awareness.

In the haṭha yoga tradition, which uses powerful techniques to induce altered states of mind, there is an emphasis on being grounded in reality through the process of dropping into the present moment by uniting the sun and the moon channels of the breath. This process, which eventually can positively enhance all aspects of your life, is not as unattainable as our minds might like to imagine. In fact, it can and does happen spontaneously all the time—even if you are not practicing yoga or meditation. Whenever you have an experience of beauty, an aesthetic awakening, or when you delight in the essence or true flavor of something, whenever you are kind or when you feel a true relationship, then the two channels of breath automatically unite. Physiologically there are a number of signals that indicate you have dropped into the calm of the central channel, but because the sensations are subtle, they may come and go unnoticed. One sign is a softening and a sense of opening up through the back of the palate. This causes the eyes to become steady yet soft, and it also stimulates the mind to become focused, but without

Nāda Tantric Body (4)

Opening the inner ear is both a beginning and an advanced practice in haṭha yoga. Listening, while allowing the eyes to gaze without the mind forming a subject or an object, gives space to the prāṇa, and to all of the elements of the body, allowing them to unfold into their true radiant form. Nāda, sometimes represented by the sound of a conch shell, is thought of as internal pure sound that absorbs the whole attention and the mind into deep samādhi, suspending all of the fluctuations of both the praṇa and the citta. Nāda is awakened by going through all of the sensation fields of the body with the fine-tooth comb of discriminating awareness. As each of the little nāḍīs within the sense fields are cleaned out, all types of inner sounds are awakened. When the attention is held in the anāhata cakra (the heart), nāda finally begins to fully absorb the mind.

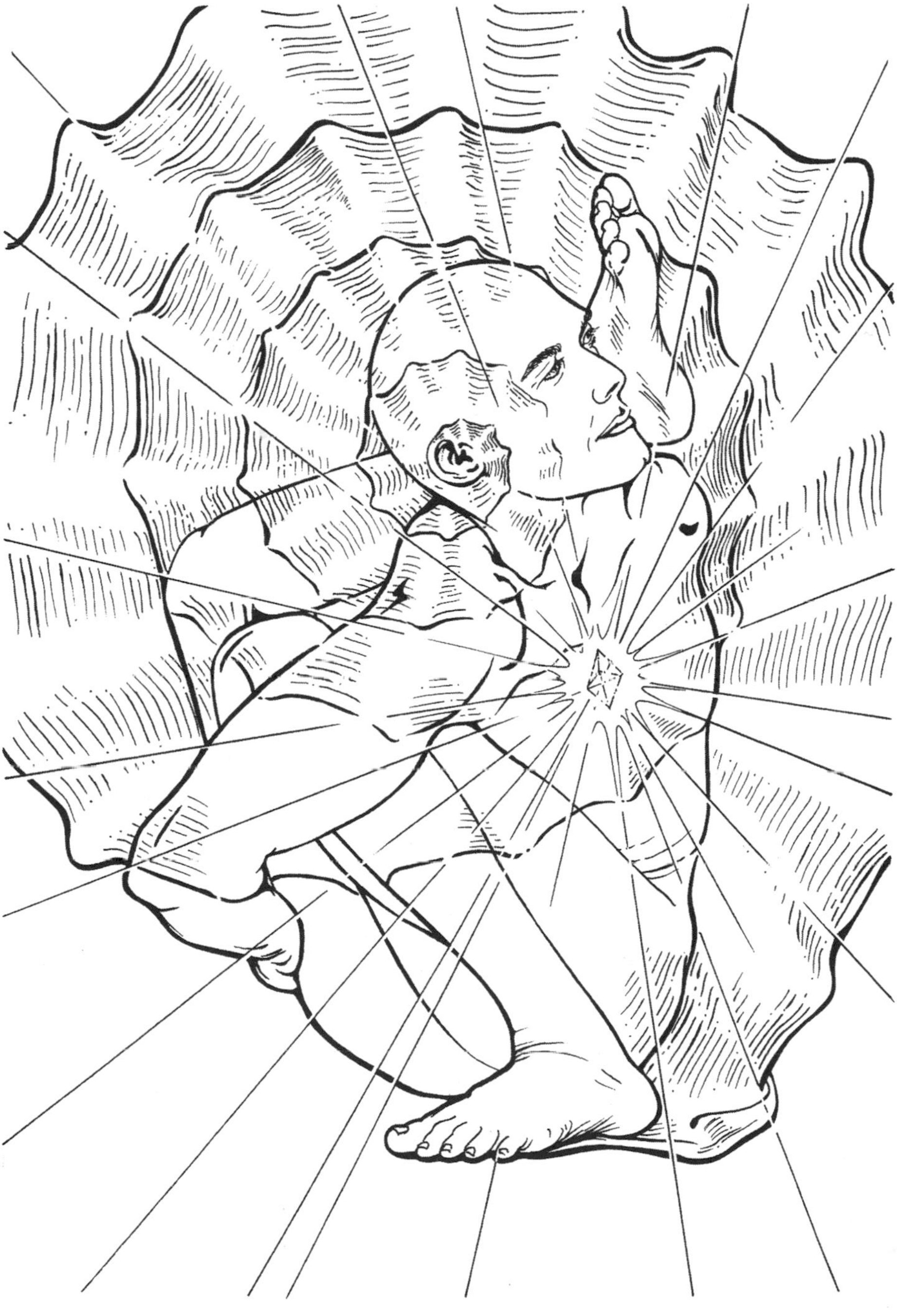

2 ends of the same stick

firm ideas, so that the mind's normal tendency to grasp the active solar attitude or the more passive lunar attitude is temporarily suspended. With practice we may notice these physiological and mental states associated with the breath dropping into the central channel as they arise, and if we stay present with the feelings while observing our ego's desire to reduce the entire experience to something we can identify and theorize about, then the yoga begins to work. We can let go and simply appreciate whatever it is that is arising, recognizing that there are always two sides to everything and that our distinct patterns of perception are usually two ends of the same stick.

Sometimes this insight into reality through an experience of the nature of the union of opposites happens spontaneously, but the awakening is also something we can nurture through the practices of yoga. For instance, we can cultivate the physiological sensations that allow the root of the palate to open. This is achieved through the simple gesture of doing nothing, of suspending technique and deferring action in an appreciation of the present moment. It is what we do whenever we say "ahhhh" and when we pay very close attention, listening, feeling, thinking about, or using any of our senses to understand something that seems interesting and fresh. If we cultivate the physiology of softening the palate, our yoga practice transforms into a fine art in which we are able to balance different ratios of our techniques—of our inward spirals and our outward spirals within a posture, for example—to find the central channel. Cultivating this refined awareness within the body, we automatically begin to balance the rooting and squeezing tendency of the apāna with the flowering and expansive pattern of the prāṇa. We equalize these aspects of breath tastefully because we know them to be the expressions of the nature of pure consciousness, of love and relationship. This automatically stimulates within us a soft, inward smile, as if we were connoisseurs of the breath. Comprehending this idea of the union of opposites initiates the process of waking up the prāṇa and inviting the kuṇḍalinī into the central axis of the body so that it can move all the way up through the crown of the head, resulting in a sense of complete release and satisfaction. It is believed that upon this full awakening, the moon at the root of the palate—which collects nectar from the thousand-petaled lotus at the crown of the head—begins to melt and to shower down nectar into all of the nāḍīs.

It may all sound rather esoteric and complicated, but that is just the mind grasping onto the idea with the desire to have the final word and a complete understanding of the concept. The actual process of this deep connection to the central channel where the prāṇa enters into the suṣumnā nāḍī, and the stunning effect this union has on both body and mind, is a completely natural occurrence if we can only step out of the way long enough to allow it to happen. If you experience kindness either through acting kindly or by receiving kindness, if you tap into a sense of compassion or mercy, what you are actually doing physiologically is releasing the soft palate, so that a drop of compassion from the vast ocean of nectar within your own heart and mind floods your awareness, and this is the essential starting point—and the necessary finishing point—of the haṭha yoga process.

4

THE ROOTS OF THE PRACTICE

> We see that all this is perishing, as these gnats, mosquitoes, and the like, the grass and the trees that grow and decay. But, indeed, what of these? There are others, superior, great warriors, . . . Kings too. . . . But, indeed, what of these? Among other things, there is the drying up of great oceans, the falling away of mountain peaks, the deviation of the pole star, the cutting of the wind-ropes (that hold the stars in their places), the submergence of the earth, the departure of the gods from their station. In such a world as this, what is the good of enjoyment of desires? For he who has fed on them is seen to return repeatedly. Be pleased, therefore, to deliver me. In this Saṁsāra (cycle of existence) I am like a frog in a waterless well. Revered Sir, you are our way, you are our way.
>
> —MAITRĪ UPANIṢAD, I.4

WITHIN THE YOGA TRADITION and Indian culture in general, the gesture of offering salutations to others—to specific gods or teachers, to physical feelings and sensations—is something that is widely used as a means of bringing awareness to direct experience in the present moment. The acknowledgments serve as reminders of the interconnected relationship of all beings and of all experiences. The salutations allow the mind to release its grip on the need to know, and at the same time, they encourage the ego to dissolve. By chanting to the "great powers of the universe," for example, we open our capacity to experience the interpenetrating meta-pattern of which we ourselves are an integral part, and also to feel the power of our breath as it relates to our mind. We are invited to look deep inside our hearts, where we start to distinguish what it is in life that really counts. Often it is not until the time of death that people return to the basic relationships in their lives as being the container for that which has held deep meaning and value for them. Chants through which we give salutations to others allow us to experience the process of appreciating that which is, rather than seeking that which we would like to be, long before we find ourselves facing our actual death. By offering our appreciation of others, we are reminded that perhaps the best way to define yoga is as a means of exploring the fundamental nature of relationship as the essence of love. In fact, it is out of this relationship to others that all of the yoga practices ultimately evolve.

In traditional yoga systems the first aspect of practice is called yama or the practice of relationship, which underscores the importance of connection to others as being integral to all expressions of yoga. The yamas are ethical principles, all of which stem from the basic tenet of ahiṁsā, or nonviolence. *Him* means "to kill" or "to harm," and *ahim* means "to not kill, to not harm." Perhaps a more accurate way of translating *ahiṁsā* is as "kindness" or "love," which could be considered the epitome of not harming; through yoga we cultivate the capacity to not harm others by offering kindness. As we dive into our yoga practice, we begin to notice that whenever we have placed another being outside of our heart—when we have behaved without kindness—we experience an underlying discontent, a deep sense of suffering that tends to color all of our experience, leaving us feeling guarded, overprotected, empty, and unfulfilled. Therefore the initial practice of yoga is to place back into our heart that which really matters, which turns out to be all sentient beings, whether they are humans or not—animals, creatures, or even imaginary life-forms. When all are located in the core of the heart, we find that the rest of the yoga practices not only clearly make sense, but that they are deeply satisfying and also that they are actually quite easy to carry out. Conversely, when we have placed even one seemingly insignificant being outside of the heart, we find that no matter what we do, the yoga practice essentially does not work; we are agitated, distracted, unhappy, or unsatisfied. So if you practice āsana or prāṇāyāma, if you twist yourself into a pretzel or you huff and you puff until you turn blue in the face, you will not be able to drop deeply inside of your own experience and truly practice yoga if you have placed even one sentient being outside of your heart. *This* is the meaning of ahiṁsā. Of course the literal meaning of nonkilling and nonharming might be interpreted to mean that a true yoga practitioner would do only good deeds and act in an absolutely sweet manner, but this is not actually so. Situations may sometimes arise in life where firm or even severe action must be taken as an act of ahiṁsā. If, for example, your child were kidnapped and beaten, the yogic response would not be to disengage and allow the situation to unfold as it might, or to try to reason with the kidnapper while your child bleeds to death on the sidewalk. Instead, ahiṁsā insinuates that one must exercise discriminative awareness in all situations that arise and then act appropriately. In this case, fitting action would be to protect your child from harm. The act of chasing the criminal down and saving your child—whatever it takes to do so—would be called for. At the same time, because the kidnapper would remain in your heart, you would act in such a way as to do the least harm possible to him or her as well. Ahiṁsā, therefore, is at the root of all relationships because as soon as we are able to reconcile our vision of others, thereby resolving our vision of what and who *we* actually are, then the yoga practices start to bear their fruit and quite naturally manifest as happiness.

The Sanskrit word for happiness is *sukha*. *Kha* means "space"; open, accommodating, radiant space. It can also mean a hole, like the hole in the center of something, and *su* means "good." The word *sukha*, therefore, can mean a good, open space in the center of something, a meaning that evolved from the idea of a chariot wheel with its hole placed precisely in the center so that when it was put to use, those in the chariot got a smooth and even ride. The word *duḥkha* is frequently translated as "suffering," but it also means a "bad hole," suggesting the idea that when the hole in a chariot's wheel was misplaced it would produce an uncomfortable, bumpy ride. When practicing, if the core of our heart is not open and truly centered, if it is not shining forth with radiance because we have closed it off to others, then our practice—and all aspects of our life—are not sukha, or happy. Instead we are filled with suffering because at the core of our being is a sense of duḥkha, or a "bad hole." If, on the other hand, we have honest relationships with others and we embrace all beings into the core of our heart, then as we wake up into the present moment we find that we are able to penetrate into the depths of our circumstances, right into the core of what we really feel, and this is the beginning of great happiness. But of course this is not always easy. The mind is programmed at all costs to avoid the heart of our circumstances, and our present moment situation in relationship to others. It almost automatically steers clear of the unknown and vehemently shies away from the raw immediacy of pure relationship with itself and with others—the reality of the present moment.

The challenge many of us find in authentic relationship is not something that is unique to our culture, nor is it the product of our times. Avoiding relationship is something that is universally experienced among human beings, and it seems to have been a problem for a very long time. The earliest stories of yoga, in the hymns of the Vedas, arose from a prehistoric, mythical time, and in poetic rhythm and metaphor they sing about the problem of relationship and the joy of its resolution in the present moment. Since the beginning of the yoga tradition many thousands, if not millions, of people have worked with this core problem of relationship (and an open, radiant heart). Countless people have cooked the idea, refined it, discussed and argued about it. They have rejected the idea, taken it up again, and they have practiced it from every conceivable angle and under every imaginable circumstance. Slowly, as schools of thought and experience evolved, the traditions of yoga have formed. Yoga, therefore, is actually not one single thing that can easily be put into words and that has an all-encompassing meaning. Instead it is a condensation and evolution of thousands of different meanings, countless experiments in consciousness, myriad of interpretations of the workings of relationship, and endless religious visions and systems, all of which have been digested and synthesized by one another. Today we are very fortunate to be able to draw on the experience of millions of people who have inquired into their hearts and, in so doing, have developed yoga as a way of penetrating into the heart of reality.

One consistent thread within all schools of yoga is that the process is initiated through a deep, visceral understanding of impermanence. It begins with an understanding that not only are our bodies extremely temporary events but so are the bodies of all other sentient beings, and that beyond that, all types of manifestations are also temporary. Quite naturally, we may be afraid to let our minds dissolve into the obvious fact that not only are *we* going to die, but our children are going to die, as are our children's children. We are all faced with the fact that our parents are going to die or have already died, as have their parents and their ancestors before them; all beings, past and future without end, are going to die. Not only that, but the circumstances in which all of these beings have lived and the environments they have created are temporary, and the very planet we are living on is an extremely impermanent event. The universe may be fourteen billion years old, but even if it endures for another trillion years, that will be just a blip in the potential of infinite time. All this is practically a truism, and we can allow our minds to unravel along these lines of thought, yet how often do we actually allow ourselves to *experience* this obvious fact? The teachings of yoga begin with the realization that we are in a situation that, from the point of view of our bodies, our circumstances, and our environment, is bleak. We are inviting disappointment and frustration as we hold on to something that is essentially made of sand. We are courting suffering. This can lead some people to think that the yoga tradition is very pessimistic or depressing because the only part of the teachings they hear is that we are all subject to birth, old age, disease, and death. In fact, even if you live a good life, eat certified organic foods, and exercise regularly, even if you do your yoga practice every day to the point that you are able to go into a deep trance at the snap of your fingers, *still* you are going to die. And in a million years, if not ten years, nobody will remember your great achievements. To the mind, which is grasping at straws, clutching for security forms that instantly dissolve, this seems like a rather negative situation to be in. But as we begin to comprehend the nature of impermanence and the universality of suffering, the effect can be quite liberating and completely grounding. We find that it is from acknowledging and assimilating the insights we have when we see that all things are temporary, that we are actually able to initiate a genuine inquiry into the practice of yoga, and more importantly, into a direct experience of the present moment. A close examination of the temporary nature of all phenomena, questioning our existence and the meaning of life, and learning to experience the actual nature of things in the present moment are the core teachings of all ancient yogic traditions.

There is a beautiful story from the time of the Buddha. He came upon a woman, Kisa Gotami, who was in a mango grove weeping with despair because her child had just died. She was so overcome by grief that she could not even grasp the truth that her child was dead. Clutching her dead child in her arms and with tear-filled eyes, she went to the Buddha and pleaded with him to help her find a miraculous medicine that would bring her child back to life. The Buddha told her to go into the village and to collect a mustard seed from each house that had not experienced the pain and suffering of having lost to death someone they loved. In the village Kisa Gotami went house to house in search of the sacred seeds that would cure her child. Of course, in doing so she discovered that every house had experienced death, that all beings who were in relationship with others had experienced the loss of someone dear to them. She went to the Buddha and became his student. He instructed her to continue meditating on the impermanent nature of all phenomena. This touching story is a vivid demonstration of the realization of the truth of impermanence, an opportunity to recognize the fact that when we die, we are not alone. All of us are dying; it is not as if everyone else is going to be staying and having a good time, carrying on and partying for all eternity.

The realization that we are all going down the tubes of time can actually be quite a cathartic release from the sense of fear and loneliness that arises when the mind first starts to contemplate impermanence. In fact, it turns out that it is this very meditation on impermanence that allows the mind to stretch itself to infinity, into the past and into the future, just as the contemplation facilitates the joining with others in an experience of true relationship. Through this insight—even in the face of death and with the knowledge that all relationships will end at some point in time—authentic connections to others are not void, nor are they perceived as a state of loneliness. Instead through the realization of impermanence, a true relationship inspires us to return home to the seed of truth that rests in the core of our heart. Ultimately, that which sounded like the most depressing news possible when we first started to contemplate it—that there is constant change and that even this glorious universe we live in is but a blip on the fabric of time—gives rise to the greatest happiness of all. Although what initially arises from a meditation on change, impermanence, and time is a brief moment of anxiety, that discomfort quickly passes if you simply stay with the presence of all that surfaces within the meditation. You find that as you become increasingly comfortable with the experience of change, the mind becomes ever more able to reframe its perceptions and to step out of itself; and then to step out of itself and reframe again, and again, and again, and again without any limitation in any direction, spontaneously igniting an incredible sense of excitement and inspiration. The Buddha taught that there are four noble truths: first, the truth of suffering; second, that there is a cause for suffering; third, that there is or can be a cessation of suffering; and fourth, that there is a path to that cessation. These truths apply directly to the path of yoga.

As an extension of the contemplation of impermanence, therefore, when you come across another person (or any sentient being for that matter) you are able to appreciate their unique yet temporary circumstances in such a way that a sincere connection with them is truly possible. When we look into each other's eyes we see that we are looking into the eyes of someone who is dying. In a sense, there is actually nothing better for your relationships—and for your own state of mind—than to realize and embrace the fact that we are all dying. Centuries ago, gaining this base understanding of impermanence was the prerequisite for learning any of the more technical aspects of yoga practice. Today with the popularization of yoga we hope that practitioners will gain a taste of this understanding through an awakened practice of postures that integrate the observation of sensation and feeling, the flow of the breath, and a pure observation of the circumstances in life.

Whether or not we practice yoga, the real problem so many of us come up against in life is that too much of the time we are busy generating theories about what is going on. We fabricate an idea about who we are today: "Today I am thin, today I am fat, today I am doing well, today I am doing badly, today I am black, I am white, I am big, I am little, I am old, I am young!" There is no shortage to the theories we generate about ourselves, others, and life itself. In fact, this is what thinking is—it is creating propositions and speculating about reality, so that we become defined by our thoughts about who we are. We describe other things by the labels we make for them, classifying them by the uses we have for them or by their function. We reduce the miracle of a tree to the name assigned to that kind of tree or to the uses we have for it, unable to appreciate the sheer presence of the tree in and of itself. Through this process of reducing the immediate experience to our thoughts about it, we become disembodied theories of ourselves and insubstantial theories of each other. We cripple ourselves, unable to touch the immediacy of life and incapable of comprehending why we are not deeply connected with others. When we reduce anything to our theories about it, we cannot really appreciate what we hear, taste, smell, feel, and see, so the magic and joy, the simplicity, and the innocence of life are lost because we are adrift in our thoughts. Stuck in thought, confusion arises and suffering begins.

Within the context of yoga, the cause of suffering is referred to as avidyā, which means "ignorance" or "to not know." Avidyā is the identification of what is eternal—true, pure life, that which is joyous and free—with what is impermanent, unconscious, and mechanical. This superimposition of what is unreal onto what is real is the same confusion we experience when we mistake what is permanent for what is impermanent. It is a form of ignorance that does not allow us to see things as they truly are. Avidyā is considered the root form of ignorance, or of not knowing, and it is deemed to be the origin of all suffering because it precludes our having genuine relationships because the confusion prevents us from appreciating others as they truly are.

In this light you could say that yoga can be summed up as one simple practice: that of observing what is actually happening in the present moment. This is not just watching sensation and feeling alone, but it is also a witnessing of the very phenomenon of ignorance (avidyā) itself. In the process of yoga we do not attempt to get rid of ignorance; we quickly discover that there is no real need of doing so. Instead we develop the art of awakening to the mental process of avidyā, by seeing that its continuous representation of one thing by another thing is inadequate and unending. We practice waking up to the fact that this habit of reducing things to our theories about them, like all else in life, dissolves as we observe it. Waking up little by little we begin to meet face-on the experience of not knowing, and we are able to accept that we do not have ultimate control over our own body, let alone the entire universe, so that as we meet the truth of impermanence, change, and time, and we find it to be remarkably exhilarating. This continuum of insight through letting the mind rest in the present moment is at the root of all yoga, which is why it is said that at first yoga seems like a poison but that it then transforms into nectar. As we begin to inquire into our existence and impermanence, observing our body and mind and then the very core of the body—all those feelings and sensations that lie along the central axis become vivid and alive. In this process of yoga, feelings of extreme fear and avoidance often arise when we first encounter change, impermanence, and the deeply rooted patterns of feeling within the body. The initial "poison" of yoga is our response to the revelation of truth, which has been avoided for years. But as we continue to practice by inviting the mind to stay with whatever is arising, rather than grasping onto pleasant perceptions and rejecting those things we see as unpleasant, then the nectar of the practice unfolds as the mind dissolves into the core of the heart, revealing the interconnected meta-pattern, the matrix of all things.

As our yoga practice evolves, our power of clear observation increases. We learn to trace continuous strings of feelings and sensations along the central axis of the body, from the pelvic floor up through the root of the navel and the core of the heart, then moving on up through the throat, behind the soft palate, between the centers of the ears, and on out through the crown of the head. When we refer to the core of the heart we mean that part of our anatomy, behind the center of the sternum, which lies on the central axis of the body, not the middle of the actual physical organ of the heart. By the root of the navel we mean behind the navel, right where the plumb line of the body and the residue of the umbilical cord connect. The center of the pelvic floor is the central tendon one-quarter inch up and in front of the anus. These points define the central channel, the suṣumnā nāḍī, and it is by meditating on this line that we refine our skill of observing subtle change within our own body and begin to intuit a deep, visceral understanding of the nature of change. Along this line we encounter feelings that are intimately connected to our theories about the world, powerful feelings that are reflected in the way we think about ourselves and others. As we develop an appreciation for perceiving things as they are, we find that meditation on the suṣumnā nāḍī becomes easier and more natural. Whenever we notice ourselves reducing things to our theories about them, we also experience uncomfortable physiological effects deep inside the core of the body, through the mirror of this sensitive, piercing channel. These subtle yet profound feelings are a physiological response to our natural tendency to short-circuit the process of change and the truth of impermanence by imposing our theories about the world onto what is actually arising. It is human nature to formulate ideas in order to understand what is arising, but when we become stuck in our own realm of name and form, created by our own mind as a means of identifying our perceptions as true, permanent, and unchanging, then we experience discomfort along the central axis of the body. We actually *feel* our own denial about the truth of impermanence right in the core of our own body. Eventually we recognize that impermanence is inseparable from those feelings of change we are experiencing, and this reveals that insight into the nature of impermanence is inseparable from an experience of having the core of the heart open and luminous. We find also that when we are aligned with the truth, the core feelings we encounter are so wonderful and sublime, *so nice,* that they are almost impossible for the mind to stay with, and that unbeknownst to us, all of our lives our own cherished mind has been devising schemes to avoid experiencing this core consciousness. It is the nature of the mind to avoid feeling these deep sensations just as it evades the core of reality and the heart of relationship. The mind shuns deeply intimate aspects of reality because such profound truth has an element of not-knowing at its foundation, and the conceptual, controlling mind avoids not-knowing like the plague. But under the right circumstances, when it feels safe and not threatened, the mind is also eager to let go of its need to know, its desire to organize, to categorize, and to define life in word and in form. The mind's initial fear of not-knowing is a taproot of the initial "poison" often experienced when starting yoga. As we stick with the simple practices, as the body's core feelings are released without obstruction, our fear of the unknown subsides and the exquisite nectar released through the practice can be experienced. The only word that truly describes these core feelings is radiance, but not our concept of radiance; rather an unknown manifestation of it that we must allow to unfold. It is the pure radiance of love. And true love, like so many acute aspects of life, is utterly dependent on surrendering theory and philosophy into the field of the great unknown.

Many thousands of years ago in India there were the ṛṣis (pronounced "rishis"), the seers, who sang the descriptive and lyrical poetry that were the hymns of the Vedas. These hymns describe the rhythms of life, the patterns and pulsations of the universe. They are prayers to God, gods, and goddesses, wrapping myths into myths and metaphors into metaphors. They proposed no one point of view, no single philosophical or theological system. In about 800 B.C.E., times changed, as they always do, and the age of philosophy began to replace the age of the gods, mythology, and poetry. This was a time in which people started to consider and discuss the patterns of *how* they were thinking about things, rather than just tolerating or not tolerating each others' myths, gods, and customs. In the philosophical age, people became interested in finding the essence of an experience in order to refine and express it more clearly and universally. This same pattern of philosophical exploration was happening all at once in Asia and in Europe, and it was particularly concentrated around ancient Greece and India. The global age of mythology—in which the myths were memorized and passed on through chanting—shifted into an age of philosophy. In India the first scriptural expressions of philosophical thought outside of the hymns of the Veda were the early Upaniṣads, which taught a group of simple unitary doctrines now know as Vedānta. *Ved* means "to know," and *anta* means the "end," so the Vedānta initially means the "end of the Veda" and esoterically implies the end of "knowing" as in a mystical experience of reality beyond the construction of thought.

The early Vedānta took terms from the Vedic hymns, such as *puruṣa, ātman,* and *Brahman,* and developed a simple path out of the delusions of a conditioned mind and into the experience of pure, awakened, open consciousness. This was said to be the real purpose of the Veda and the ultimate purpose of human life. The ordinary meaning of the word *puruṣa* is "man," as in human. The ordinary meaning of *ātman* is "self" as in myself, and Brahman has always referred to the all-pervasive, ever-opening radiance that is pure being. The sages of the Upaniṣads taught that the true self is not any of the localized, temporary sheaths that we mistake it to be; rather it is pure, unconditioned awareness itself, identical to the Brahman. Even more important (and here is the slippery counterthought), the ātman is not a separate thing from the world we experience. When we are seeing this world, this experience clearly, we are seeing ātman. When seen incorrectly due to ignorance, or avidyā, we see separate and unconnected things making up the world. This early teaching of nondualism is best conveyed by the texts themselves:

> For where there is duality as it were, there one sees the other, one smells the other, one tastes the other, one speaks to the other, one hears the other, one thinks of the other, one touches the other, one knows the other. But where everything has become just one's own self [ātman], by what and whom should one see, by what and whom should one smell, by what and whom should one taste, by what and to whom should one speak, by what and whom should one hear, by what and of whom should one think, by what and whom should one touch, by what and whom should one know? By what should

> one know him by whom all this is known? That self [ātman] is (to be described as) not this, not this.
>
> (*Bṛhad Āraṇyaka Upaniṣad*, IV.5.15)

From this declaration that the ātman is "not this, not this" arises the early form of dialectical thinking that serves to continuously take us deeper into experience by not allowing us to cling to partial or incomplete versions of the whole. In Sanskrit "not this, not this" is *neti neti*, words that actually make a pleasant chant, adding on as many netis as you like, enjoying the reverberation of the sound and occasionally drawing your mind back into the meaning that all of this is "not this," not what you think. The neti neti methodology has been called by modern thinkers "negative dialectics." Such a cheery, warm name has given many contemporaries the wrong idea about the early yoga philosophy (and even some early philosophers had the same misconception). Not used to metaphysical thinking, some consider yoga philosophy to be negative, gloomy, pessimistic, and even depressing. When grounded in the fact of impermanence, however, yogins find negative dialectics to be as sweet as honey and as bright as sunshine, since negative dialectics allow us to let go of temporary conceptual divisions as they spread through ever finer layers of our thinking. Teachings and philosophical statements are often misunderstood and taken out of context when first heard. Yoga students are often bewildered by the discussions and arguments that go back and forth within and between schools of yoga, as we misunderstand each other and ourselves rather than observing the phenomena in all of their layers. The arguments, misunderstandings, and constant changes of viewpoint and definition have their own importance and beauty.

The early Upaniṣads are beautiful expressions of the truth, but their ideas had not yet matured in the fires of debate and questioning that inevitably occur when you meet someone from another system or from a different culture or religion. The early philosophical thinking found in the Upaniṣads was first condensed and developed into what is called the Sāṁkhya system by a sage named Kapila in about 600 B.C.E., just before the time of the Buddha. The system was later refined and placed in the form the *Sāṁkhya Kārikā* by the philosopher Īśvara Kṛṣṇa. It is through Sāṁkhya terminology that most different philosophical schools of yoga and Vedānta, and even various systems of Buddhism, have based their arguments. To understand yoga it is important to appreciate and to study Sāṁkhya even if we do not agree with all of its propositions. The word *Sāṁkhya,* which literally means "to count or innumerate," is in one sense essentially a listing of all of the different things that we encounter in both our external and internal experience. The system describes the layers of reality that are nested one within the other—a hierarchical ordering of sorts—aspects of which we touch in the direct experience of meditating, making it simultaneously a psychological and a philosophical system. Sāṁkhya is primarily a tool that explains and illuminates the experience of close observation of the very process of life, while also explaining philosophically who we are, what the world is, and how the cosmos might be structured.

It is very important to realize when looking at any of these early philosophical systems, including Sāṁkhya, that though they present a philosophical doctrine, they are intended to be psychological tools that provide a view of what the immediate experience might have been of the sage who was writing the text. So it is good to approach a system like this with an open mind, an open heart, and with a grain of salt. In fact, while studying yoga in general, and yoga philosophy in particular, it is very important to give yourself license to entertain different ideas. There is no obligation at all that you must believe or buy into the ideas presented in a text. The intention of the original philosophers was quite the contrary; it was that you would learn to think for yourself so you could experience reality as it is. When studying philosophy you will always get far more out of it if you yourself go deeply into whatever thought is being presented, rather than simply swallowing the philosophical propositions without question, allowing someone else to do the thinking and experiencing for you. You should never accept any philosophy simply because someone else has said it is so, and this experimental characteristic of good philosophy has endured to this day within parts of the yoga tradition.

Sāṁkhya philosophy is based on a dualistic axiom that draws a line splitting what we believe to be the totality of the universe into two very clear categories. One category is called puruṣa and the other prakṛti. *Prakṛti* means "creative energy." *Puruṣa,* though literally meaning "man" or "human," refers to the seer or the one who is experiencing the universe, and in this sense puruṣa is you. The split differentiates and makes sense of the experience of consciousness by defining as two separate categories that which is the true self and of true value (puruṣa), and the endless world of forms that are the content of experience (prakṛti). The nature of puruṣa is that it is the seer, the witness; it is pure consciousness. The nature of prakṛti is that it is the seen, the object of awareness. Prakṛti, then, is everything that is presented as a limited form or a limited pattern, gross or subtle, as well as the substratum or cause that is behind whatever is presented. In other words, prakṛti is anything and everything. You, the puruṣa, perceive small corners or bits of prakṛti as whatever is presented in your awareness. So the object—be it a cloud in the sky, a thought, an emotion, a physical sensation, or an everyday object like a teakettle—is the seen, it is prakṛti. Puruṣa, the seer, is simply pure awareness, pure consciousness. This distinction between puruṣa and prakṛti, the underlying structural understanding that all we encounter in life is the seen, is the foundational tenant of Sāṁkhya. The idea seems simple enough, but when you think more deeply about the idea, it becomes quite slippery, incredibly difficult for the mind to keep hold of, because it requires the mind to examine itself. From the perspective of Sāṁkhya, the mind's own perceptions, its own conclusions about what it is perceiving (for example, thinking that it understands the basic definition of Sāṁkhya as a dualistic system that defines puruṣa and prakṛti), even an idea of the person who believes himself or herself to be at the helm of the mind, the one who is doing all of the perceiving (you)—all of those things are aspects of prakṛti. So understanding the difference between prakṛti and puruṣa can be very confusing at first, because everything that we experience in the outer world as well as everything in our inner world is prakṛti. The tangible things we encounter, like another person or a stop sign, as well as things we encounter within our imagination, including all of the ideas and subtle feelings that we might have about the puruṣa or consciousness itself, are prakṛti. Puruṣa is strictly pure consciousness, pure perception. Once puruṣa is recognized, identified, named, at that instant those labels, images, and feelings form as prakṛti. Puruṣa cannot be cognized or re-cognized as an object or thing at all, which is what makes the Sāṁkhya system so confounding and difficult to understand.

The most popular metaphor for the puruṣa-prakṛti relationship (or perhaps more accurately, their lack of relationship) is that of the sun and a flower. The sun, puruṣa or pure consciousness, simply shines. This sunshine causes the flower—which is the perennial symbol of prakṛti—to open and to turn toward the sun. Here the metaphor is not really dualistic, because the sun has some influence on the flower. Unavoidably, some quality is being given to puruṣa that inspires, wills, loves, or stimulates prakṛti. The mystical experience that was described poetically in the Vedas, and then philosophically in the ātman-Brahman teaching of the early Upaniṣads, is defined in the Sāṁkhya system as when the puruṣa simply sees prakṛti as prakṛti without identifying with and latching onto any identification with what is seen and without naming the perception. Prakṛti simply *is* creative energy. In fact, any of us at any time could engage in a completely proper Sāṁkhya meditation by just acknowledging that whatever we think, feel, see, touch, smell, taste, or hear—that any and every *thing* we are capable of perceiving is prakṛti. A constant sense of discriminating awareness that all layers of the perceived are only prakṛti allows the complete unfolding of the flower of prakṛti. However, it is very difficult for the mind (filled with idolatrous images of puruṣa) to hold the insight that prakṛti is a unified, hierarchical field of creative energy, empty of puruṣa and without connection to puruṣa. To complicate matters, in order to make such a meditation truly fall in line with the deeper intention of the Sāṁkhya system, we must understand that our mental mantras or the phrase "all is prakṛti" is, in and of itself, also prakṛti.

Though the Sāṁkhya system can sometimes seem confusing, it essentially offers encouragement to really look when we are looking. Within the Sāṁkhya model, when we are able to observe our present experience as being prakṛti, then we can finally suspend the infinitely exhausting process of theorizing and philosophizing about our experience. We can drop fully into our immediate experience, and *this* is the foundation of all mystical experience. We see right from the beginning that the Sāṁkhya system (and in fact all of the early yoga philosophies) is an attempt to expose false self or false puruṣa. These systems are vehicles that are to be abandoned just at the right moment so that the vehicle itself becomes part of the fuel for the process of awareness rather than the focus of our awareness. To the beginner the Sāṁkhya system appears to be an uncompromising dualistic system in which puruṣa is totally separate from prakṛti. As novices we might think that the puruṣa is liberated when we imagine the distinction between a solid, ego-like, human-shaped puruṣa floating above an elemental, dead, mechanical, and always shifting prakṛti. But this is a beginner's theory and is part of the mind's attempt to categorize, label, and solidify the two distinct parts of the dualism so that one side is bad (temporary) and the other side is good (permanent). The actual dualistic axiom of Sāṁkhya works to constantly deconstruct any image or idea of puruṣa. Puruṣa is not a thing, not a noun, not a verb, and not even a function. That prakṛti cannot define or pin down puruṣa keeps prakṛti open, moving, and fresh. Perhaps the reason Sāṁkhya philosophers stuck to this apparent dualism, at no point conceding the obvious fact that prakṛti and puruṣa are not two separate "things," is that they wanted us to be able to experience even the most subtle states of mind as being empty of ego, empty of self, empty of puruṣa. If we capitulate too soon in our understanding and say, "Oh yes, puruṣa and prakṛti are ultimately the same thing," then we inevitably wind up identifying with some aspect or layer of the mind right in the midst of an arising experience, at which point selfness, separateness, puruṣa-ness gets projected into the woven fabric of prakṛti. In this way we establish ego, which short-circuits the actual mystical experience and derails us from having a truly deep insight into the actual nature of consciousness.

Within the Sāṁkhya system it is said that the ground from which the universe of our experience unfolds is called mūla prakṛti. *Mūla* means "root," and *prakṛti* of course means "creative energy." In this original state, prakṛti is said to be like a clear, bright, empty mirror that simply reflects pure living consciousness. Balanced, fully integrated mūla prakṛti reflects contentless consciousness; it reflects only puruṣa. Any imbalance—a seed, a flaw—makes the root prakṛti generate the world and our experiences of it. The basic building blocks of the Sāṁkhya universe, the cosmos of our direct experience, are called the three guṇas. *Guṇa* means a "strand" or a "rope," and it is said, within the Sāṁkhya system that these three strands braided together generate the process of prakṛti, the process of constant change, continual transformation and evolution. Everything at all levels of manifestation is said to be a different combination of these three basic energetic threads of creation. The term *guṇa* has been interpreted in many different ways. Some define the guṇas according to their separate physical characteristics—one strand being bright and balanced, one having movement and interaction, and one being fixed and full of inertia. However, if we look at the guṇas as merely physical properties that we experience in the outside universe, then we tend to exclude the more important subjective psychological properties they each have as part of our feelings within our internal landscape. A more complete and accurate understanding of the guṇas connects the inner world of our perception, thought, and mind state with the outer physical world.

The three guṇas are sattva, rajas, and tamas. Sattva is associated with principles of synthesis, harmony, knowledge, intelligence, happiness, and goodness. Rajas is the energy of antithesis, passion, activity, motion, desire, and sorrow. Tamas is the quality of thesis, inertia, fixity, dullness, darkness, illusion. All three are constantly in dynamic tension with one another. Their relationship is somewhat like an ongoing game of rock, paper, scissors, because in all that occurs in life, one guṇa—one of the strands—gets on top, but no one remains on top since none of the guṇas are of fixed substance. The guṇas, therefore, are a means of describing the process of evolution or change and impermanence. Every experience we have is composed of the transformation of the three guṇas, and it is said that the activities of the guṇas are the unfolding of eternal time itself.

Tamas can be understood to be the past, that which has been determined and is history; it is the objective situation, the given, your lot in life. Tamas refers to all aspects of experience that have a predominantly fixed or tamasic quality to them. One way to understand tamas is as that which is given to us with no effort. Rajas can be understood to be more closely associated with the future; it is desire, projection, externalization. Sattva is the synthesis of the position of tamas and the counterposition of rajas. It is ultimately the understanding of selflessness and is considered to be the present moment with the quality of awakening; it is the process of consciousness unfolding. Sattva transcends the tension between past and future, between what has happened and what the mind projects as the possibilities of what could happen. It can be cultivated to the point of such clarity that it becomes like a clear mirror for the light of puruṣa. When the processes of prakṛti are observed without interference, sattva is the naturally occurring state of affairs.

As the threads of sattva, rajas, and tamas intertwine within our ever-changing experience we find our perceptions and our moods dominated by one or another of the three guṇas. Often we find ourselves in a sattvic mood, and in that state of being we tend to do things that in turn are labeled as sattvic: we eat sattvic foods, those that have a balancing effect on the body, or we engage in sattvic activities, like being kind. When we are first in a sattvic mood our perceptions are clear and bright. The feelings of joy, love, compassion, empathy are right up near the surface of our awareness, and virtually everything we experience stimulates one of these "good" and satisfying feelings. Consequently we behave, think, and react in ways that reflect this sattvic state of being. But after some time spent in a sattvic mood—and it can be a long or a very short period of time—we become desensitized to the joyful stimulation of the sattvic state, and usually without even being aware of it, we reduce the good state to a formula or image and begin to drift off into a state of complacency, dullness, boredom, and inertia; the state of tamas sets in. Our senses become lifeless, we are drawn to lackluster activities, for example, sticking to routines or eating foods that make us feel thick and heavy, and we become sluggish, unmotivated, or uninspired. Again after some time (if we are lucky) this dull state of being becomes intolerable and it stimulates the rajasic guṇa to kick in; we become very eager to do things, almost anxious to act. Passionate or angry, our actions are fast and not always well thought through, and we are drawn to nourish the body in ways that reinforce our ability to stay zealous—like having another cup of coffee. This rajasic quality breaks up the dullness and the inertia that set in when we fell into a tamasic state. It can draw us back into a sattvic state if we are able to remain fully conscious and harness our rajasic energy skillfully, funneling it into a state of calm, clear thinking and action. But if we remain rajasic for too long, we become imbalanced and maybe even aggressive, unthoughtful, attached to the formulas of opposition, and ungrounded, which eventually results in burnout that propels us back into a tamasic state.

The effect of this ever-changing, cyclical pattern of the guṇas is that we are always in transition. The yoga practices teach us to cultivate awareness in all of these different states of being so that we remain fluid, alert, and able to transition from one to the next skillfully. We learn to do this by remembering that the nature of a harmonized, sattvic state is similar to a piece of fruit: it will ripen and become heavenly just before it starts to overripen and rot. But unlike a piece of fruit, our states of being are completely renewable; the sattvic feeling of contentment becomes a vibrant rajasic state of being, which (if we stay alert) again becomes sattvic. Of course, once again after some time, the sattvic state becomes too peaceful, decays into a dull or tamasic state, which is finally interrupted by a burst of rajasic energy, and the cycle continues. This pattern of the guṇas occurs not only in our moods; as is pointed out in the system of Sāṁkhya, it is considered to be the underlying process of change in all perceivable experience inside and outside of our body.

Even though the sattvic state is harmonized, compassionate, selfless, and joyful, and it might seem that the "goal" of the practice of yoga is to make you purely sattvic, paradoxically this is not so. For a state to be truly sattvic, it must have at least in its background the elements of tamas and rajas, and it must occur spontaneously. If you become attached to the idea that being in a constant sattvic state is most desirable, and you then try to become sattvic, either you will wind up rajasic in your pursuit of sattva or you will become upset at the inevitable decay of your happy sattvic state into a sleepy, dull, fixed tamasic state. In either case you will suffer deeply. You may not recognize yourself as being in a constant state of attempting to sculpt all situations as you strive to be sattvic, but if you do not fully cherish and look upon with equanimity the other states of being, you will never be truly sattvic, completely fulfilled. It is common for beginning yoga students to become so attached to the idea of a sattvic state that they become stuck pushing or pulling on the tamasic state of mind that is at the edges of sattva. The apparent paradox in this situation arises because if you are not a little attracted to a sattvic state when you practice yoga or sit down to meditate, then you have no motivation to practice at all. If you are not on some level yearning to have a good practice, then there will be no practice at all and no chance to observe how silly the mind is when making goals for practicing. Practice exposes how the mind works through both useful and hurtful ego games. When the mind creates an ideal of the sattvic practice, then instead of truly being present with experience as it spontaneously arises and transforms, you compare everything to the ideal, making it impossible to observe any uncomfortable tamasic state. You find yourself in a rajasic state; your practice is filled with grasping, frustration, and a need to achieve the ideal. It is ironic that we can understand the cyclical nature of the guṇas within all experience, but that we so often grasp onto the desire for a sattvic state. An overestimation of our own purity makes us reject and condemn any useful rajas in us, so that we do not even notice it when we become stuck in a tamasic state of being. Herein lies the paradox that surrounds the guṇas. We find that the practice of yoga frequently presents paradoxes (philosophically, emotionally, mentally, and physically) that place us in double binds that seem ironic and impossible to navigate. If we are fortunate enough to be in a sattvic and alert state when one of these paradoxes arises, then we can see that such double binds are inevitable and that they are actually at the root of some of the great depth of life's experience, and perhaps we can also even see that they are a little bit humorous.

It is possible for the mystical experience to occur through our insight into one of these paradoxical situations, when we truly comprehend that all experience is simply the three guṇas acting on each other. This can occur if, when a happy or a sattvic state arises, that very state becomes the object of our attention. We can witness the state as it naturally disintegrates into dullness, but we observe the disintegration, we do not identify with the breakdown or the tamasic state itself. Instead we are able to observe this shifting of the guṇas as the natural pattern of change. Then when the passion of the rajasic state naturally arises, when ideas surface that start to stir things up again, at that point we understand that what is happening is simply the guṇas acting on the guṇas. In this way we are able to appreciate the process of life happening, and there is an actual opportunity for the spontaneous awakening of a mystical experience. If, on the other hand, we do not understand that all experience is the intertwining of these three braids of prakṛti and that change is the natural outcome of that interdependent relationship, then we become extremely attached at certain phases of our experience and repulsed at other junctures, which eventually leads us to regret the very process of transformation itself.

5

Buddhi and Context

One way to look at the Sāṁkhya universe as it blossoms out of the effect of the guṇas interacting on each other and on all things, a universe that revolves around the interplay of the prakṛti and the puruṣa, is to compare it to a dark chocolate confection with a creamy filling. The further you go into that piece of candy the sweeter it gets, and at the very center is the essence, an intensely delightful core. In the middle of the Sāṁkhya universe is the most lovable spot, a seat of clear intelligence where the higher sattvic functions come to balance. In the absolute center of this seat is the resting point or gateway of the puruṣa. All of this can be visualized as a maṇḍala or a yantra representing the Sāṁkhya universe with all of life, experience, all mind states, and each of the guṇas vacillating around the exterior, pulsating in toward the very center resting point of puruṣa. The part that is closest to the center and to puruṣa is called the buddhi. The word *buddhi,* derived from the verbal root *budh*, "to awaken," is best translated as "intelligence." It is the principle of awakening, the ability to step outside of a framework, as if we were waking up from a dream. Buddhi is the first thing to evolve out of the essence of the root mūla prakṛti, and is often symbolized as being like a creeper, wrapping itself around puruṣa, just as a vine entwines a post. In another sense, buddhi is like a close cousin of both puruṣa and prakṛti—the missing link that ties together the vast open and pure quality of puruṣa with the more specific, object-centered quality of prakṛti. Buddhi is the very nature of the sattva guṇa, and it is perhaps the most important (though possibly also the most difficult) aspect of the Sāṁkhya system to understand.

The buddhi can be defined as the "context maker" because true intelligence is the ability to discover the real meaning of things by linking them into their contexts. Buddhi receives input from the senses, the mind, and memory, and then draws the outline or frame of that given input in order to put it in context. The Sāṁkhya system teaches that our experience is both given to us (in a passive realistic sense) and subjectively created (in an idealistic sense). Buddhi sees relationships between objects; it reveals their background and allows that knowledge to continuously interface for whatever purpose the buddhi chooses to serve. In the long run it is the buddhi that actually allows you to understand and to fully experience you as you: puruṣa as puruṣa. When integrated and awakened, "she" (or buddhi in feminine personification) exists for the purpose of revealing puruṣa, as a striker exists for a bell or as a lover for the beloved. Her purpose, however, is more often diverted toward the ego or what is called the false puruṣa. Buddhi's potentially brilliant functioning becomes dull and clogged by deeply held needs and fears that come from a basic ignorance that sees some parts of prakṛti as separate and permanent objects. Splayed out by visions of myriad sense objects, buddhi keeps becoming fixed by the contexts it creates or by the relationships it discovers between the forms. When the mind latches onto the partial meanings derived through its clogged up "context maker," it easily loses sight of the fact that in every instant of every experience it is only the guṇas that are acting on the guṇas. Waking up, cleaning up the buddhi function, therefore necessitates a continuous reevaluation of context, a reframing of our frames of reference, an ongoing, working meditative intelligence so that we can comprehend that everything we perceive is prakṛti.

We can understand this complex core principle of the Sāṁkhya system through our own physical experience within our yoga practice. For example, it is easy to admit that you do not have complete control over which sensations are being presented to you—there might be a sensation in your quadriceps, a pain in your shoulder, a pinching in your abdomen, or a sense of stretching in the skin in front of your heart. However, the true insight and freedom within any posture actually comes from being able to observe the sensations, whatever they are, as they arise. In the same way, insight into pure consciousness, into puruṣa, lies quite simply in your ability to intelligently stay with the content that is being presented to you (in this case the feelings, thoughts, and sensations as they arise in your āsana practice). If you (false puruṣa) can then step out of the way, your own buddhi, your own intelligence, like a focused lens, will keep seeing through, balancing, and opening the contextual background of whatever you are observing, so that the mind does not jump away. Through yoga, the buddhi is said to become purified, meaning that as we practice, the intelligence no longer gets derailed by the mind but sees through the labels and thoughts about the particular content that is being presented. If we look at the Sāṁkhya universe as being an unfolding flower, then the puruṣa sits right within the buddhi at the center of that flower, either caught in the drama of interfacing identity with the flower or basking in the clear light, the mirror of the buddhi's integrated, balanced, intelligence. In fact, the second and the tenth chapters of the *Bhagavad Gītā* describe yoga as being buddhi yoga—the yoga of pure intelligence.

The next thing that evolves out of buddhi is called ahaṁkāra—the I-maker or the ego function. Though essential to establishing form and organisms in this world, it can become the stem of endless suffering and loneliness. Within the Sāṁkhya system ahaṁkāra is considered to be a sacred process that occurs within prakṛti. It has been called the cit-acit granthi, the knot that ties together that which is cit or pure consciousness (puruṣa) with that which is acit or unconsciousness (prakṛti). The knot forms as a mysterious sense of a subjective "I," which continuously collects images, theories, and beliefs about itself as separate from others and from its environment. It arises from basic ignorance, the confusion of puruṣa with prakṛti. It causes us to quickly create subject-object relationships in the sense fields by endowing countless small sections of prakṛti with self, thereby pulling objects out of their backgrounds. The ahaṁkāra, the ego, then accepts or rejects the objects according to its perceived need to protect and maintain itself as a separate organism, blocking the inherent flow of information within the buddhi that would lead to truer perception and insight. This confusion of ego, this blocking of the intelligence of interdependence, is still ultimately the guṇas acting on the guṇas and is every bit as sacred as any of the other manifestations of prakṛti, any other perception or insight, and any of the other processes of the buddhi. In fact the ego is essential to life because it allows us to at least temporarily draw boundaries and identify particular things—this body, this thought, this object—as separate from everything else.

To understand the importance of ahaṁkāra, imagine it as a seed. Generally a seed has a hard outer surface, which keeps it separated from what is outside of its exterior shell. At a certain point, if it is a lucky seed, it falls into the ground, and with the presence of moisture, the outer casing begins to soften until it is sufficiently supple and becomes porous. At this point there is communication between the inside of the seed—which has information—and the external environment. It is that exchange of information that stimulates the growth of the seed so that transformation, life itself, can begin to occur. Likewise, we have an ego that is like a shell that allows our potential, the manifestation of our truest self, to develop. At certain junctures of interaction with others or with the environment—which are usually points of illumination, transformation, or insight—our ego becomes porous. If we stay present with the process of change that we are encountering, and if we stay tuned into the process of the guṇas acting on the guṇas, then we are carefully able to let go of those things we identify as ourselves and release the perceptions that falsely or partially identify others and other things as separate for us and from each other. In this way we are able to assimilate things that lie beyond our immediate system, whether they are outside our philosophical system or the physical system of our body. This assimilation process allows us to experience transformation or growth, and in witnessing our own process of change there is the possibility of discovering what we *really* are deep at the core. Yoga actually makes the ego function porous. Periodic letting go of ego positions and images keeps the function useful and healthy, allowing insights to occur. Having no ego function would mean the death of our physical organism, but learning to become fluid within our ego system leads to insight. The ego, the ahaṁkāra, is useful in that it always gives us stuff to let go of. It is sacred in that when its contracting function arises in us or in others, it should be observed as it is.

Another function of the ahaṁkāra is to facilitate a shift of focus away from pure consciousness by turning the activity of the buddhi outward in a relentless attempt to create a false self, or a false puruṣa. This process is represented in the myth of Rāma, in which Rāma's beloved consort Sītā was captured by the demon Rāvaṇa, who carried her away to Śrī Lanka. This event set off the yogic cycle of activity that is part of the ancient epic tale the *Rāmāyaṇa*. In the story the demon Rāvaṇa is the ego, the false puruṣa, who steals the buddhi, or Sītā, away from pure consciousness, Rāma, the true puruṣa. Rāma then enlists the son of the wind god, Hanūmān who represents prāṇa, and which cleans and integrates the buddhi. Hanūmān steals Sītā back and burns down the city, which represents the structures around the inflated ego, Rāvaṇa. Ultimately Rāma defeats Rāvaṇa in an incredible battle, and this defeat necessitates all of the other events that happen within the story and which are symbolic of the yoga process. The story should be read by all students of yoga

The next layer that evolves within Sāṁkhya after buddhi and the ahaṁkāra is called manas, or "mind." Manas is considered simply to be the organizer of perception. Depending on circumstances, it gives attention to particular feelings, thoughts, and sensations that come into our awareness while it completely ignores other things that arise. We are constantly surrounded by a sea of information that reaches us through the senses, and at the same time, we are continually creating stories and hypotheses about these things on an internal—often subconscious—level based on our theories. The vital function that is served by manas is to select and filter the onslaught of information that our awareness is picking up. Manas is said to have two basic functions: saṅkalpa and vikalpa. *Kal* means "to imagine," while *san* means "together" and *vi* means "divided." *Saṅkalpa,* therefore, means to imagine or to construct things into a whole, to unify them. The process takes a collection of various things that appear to be separate and recognizes their commonality, unifying them and putting them all together into one category, one box. At this point the second function of manas steps in; turning the mind around and practicing vikalpa, it divides those very same things back up into separate units or subcategories. So the mind will put everything together into a nice, neat, whole, unified package, and then it will dump everything back out again. All this is to say that the mind has a capacity and a propensity to make both a divided construction and a unified construction; it accepts things and then turns right around and rejects those very things—all of this based on the ego function: "This is something I can use. This is something I can recognize. I will take this in. This is useless, and I will reject it." It is at this level of manas where the internal world of ideas and feelings meets the outer world of actual sense perceptions. It is where the rubber meets the road. For example, if we are holding a piece of fruit, a practical decision must be made on whether to eat it or not. With data from the senses we move back and forth from the senses to the buddhi through the organizing function of the manas, judging ripeness, odor, and texture against internally stored past experiences, hunger rating, food theories, beliefs, and so on, until we finally make the choice whether or not to eat the fruit.

Yoga is a very grounding art because through it we work with and accommodate the innate functions and shortcomings of buddhi, ahaṁkāra, and manas against the feedback of the outer world. The intelligence is purified through the practice, and the ego then becomes porous, allowing the manas, or the more mechanical and immediate function of the mind, to begin to work with clarity. Through the practice we are able to pay attention to the actual feedback we get from the outside world, and at the same time we can balance this input with the desires, constructs, and imagination of our inner world. Bringing these two worlds into balance helps us to come into the present moment, at which point we are considered to be grounded. But the deep effects of the yoga practice do not stop there. From ahaṁkāra and manas we start to unfold the real forms, sensations, and objects of our experience, which lie in what are called the five elements (space, air, fire, water, and earth). These five elements are interdependent transformations of the three guṇas—sattva, rajas, and tamas—and they occur not only in the outside world as objects but also in our internal world as current, remembered, and imagined sense perceptions, that is, touch, smell, taste, sounds, shapes, colors, textures, and so on. Even our most subtle feelings, our most sublime internal sensations, or whatever our most graphic vision might be, all of this has as its content some blending of the five elements. Every perception, each sensation we can experience, is actually composed of a unique pattern of these elements. The five elements unfold out of each other hierarchically from subtle to gross. The gross are always considered to be condensations of *all* of the subtle layers that have come before them. In fact, without the five elements, there is nothing for the manas, the buddhi, and the ahaṁkāra to do!

The first of the elements is called *ākāśa* or "sky." Ākāśa is the quality of nonobstructive, radiant space, which is said to correspond to hearing. In a way you can experience space when you "simply listen" because you are hearing, but you are not naming, categorizing, drawing conclusions about, or identifying the sounds you perceive. You merely experience sound vibration within space. In fact, you are also experiencing yourself, because your thoughts are not creating any form of obstruction to anything that might appear in the space of your listening. Just like the sky does not obstruct clouds—they are free to arise, to transform, or to blow away altogether—so too when you simply listen you are not obstructing the sounds that arise. Through ākāśa, meditation on the other elements can begin to occur because we give space to those elements to be as they are. From ākāśa unfolds *vāyu,* or the element of air. Like the wind, vāyu describes motion through both inner and outer space and establishes the beginning of distinctive form in which location is defined, and then movement from that point to another occurs. Vāyu corresponds to the sense of touch and is intimately related to prāṇa, the substratum of the actual process of thought. Unfolding from vāyu is *tejas,* or fire, a hot, upward-expanding opening movement. Tejas is light and deals with the sense of sight. From fire comes the element *apas,* or water, which is representative of a downward contracting flow and is said to correspond to the sense of taste. It describes external movement of actual water in the outside world as well as the sensation of downward, waterlike internal movement. From apas, the final and most gross element of all is earth, or *pṛthivī,* which is complete cohesion. Pṛthivī results from having packed everything together into a solid mass that totally obstructs movement. This final element, pṛthivī, is said to deal with smell, and to a certain extent it is the complete opposite of ākāśa, the sky element. Pṛthivī represents the quality of tamas guṇa, in which things are completely fixed or solid. Though it might seem undesirable to find yourself in the tamas guṇa, because it is associated with dullness, tamas also has the characteristic of being the foundational and historical aspect of things. For example, a geologist studying the earth and its rock formations and mountains is dealing with something that has a very deep history to it from which life continually pours forth. When you contemplate the realm of geology you may study what seem like static aspects of the universe—rock formations—but when you look closely you realize that you are seeing a stop frame along a continuum of change through an incredibly long period of time. Through geology you can start to really comprehend what time means, which is one of the glorious things about paying attention to anything that is historical; it makes our imaginative world seem almost trivial. The same is true when you contemplate space. If you go out on a clear night and look up at the stars with a telescope at distant galaxies, you get the nauseating feeling and the idea that there is really no end to that space—it is immensely vast. But if the sky were blank, if there were no stars and galaxies out there, you would simply have a vague notion that what you were looking at is vast and expansive. As soon as any form of one or a combination of the other elements appears as a defined field, the space itself shifts because it is the form that actually provides context and a way of appreciating the unlimited, accommodating dimensions of the space. Likewise the five elements complement and give perspective to each other. We experience these elements as different modes of structure, processes, and movements in the outside world, and in the inside world we experience them as different qualities of internal sensation. So when one of the elements is dominant within our mind, then that means we are appreciating internally particular patterns of movement and relationship that are associated with that element.

The distinct qualities of the five elements can be used for focusing the mind in meditation on any one of them. Remembering that the elements are hierarchical and that they unfold from each other (from ākāśa to earth), we see that one element helps in the experiencing of another one inside or around the body. Ākāśa gives space through listening to all of the elements. Centered around the throat, it allows you to feel the body as being open, infinite space or sky in all directions. This spacious attention allows you to feel the touch of air or vāyu around the heart area shifting, rolling, and flowing freely as it redefines the sense of the open sky of the ākāśa. The sense of vāyu makes it easy to define from the roots of the navel up around the edges of the diaphragm the strong spreading and rising movement associated with fire, tejas. By contrast, underneath the fire, below the navel and into the inner thighs, is the distinct opposite: the cool, downward flow of water, apas. Water is the best way to find the earth in the pelvic floor, sitting bones, backs of legs. Let water flow freely down, and it will eventually get the earth to respond, stopping, channeling, and containing the water.

The five elements are experienced both internally and externally through the five senses, or indriyas. The five senses are like fields in which sense objects or sensations arise and fall like flowers in a meadow. The sense fields themselves are experienced by yogins in meditation as the five tanmātras of each element or sense. *Tanmātra* means "moment of that-ness" and refers ultimately to the open quality of sensation when it is experienced without any overlay of concept. This open quality allows a spreading of the awareness out from any particular sensation point into the background field of potential sensation points.

We have now unfolded the basic Sāṁkhya world from the inside out and have just given hints about how meditation and yoga practice will allow us to trace our direct sense experiences back in through the various layers of mind and buddhi to eventually watch prakṛti fulfill her ultimate purpose of revealing puruṣa. A quick summary of Sāṁkhya might go like this: the mysterious pure consciousness, puruṣa, somehow interfaces with the buddhi, which generates an ego-making function. This manifests the dividing-constructing and symbol-making mind, which takes in and organizes data from the senses and sends actions and reactions back out into the world through organs of action like the hands. The world is composed of the five gross elements and other puruṣa-prakṛti cognitive systems called other sentient beings. All of this is an interweaving of the energetic strands of the three guṇas, strands that stretch as a unified whole, a tapestry or network of time itself.

When learning about Sāṁkhya philosophy, it is important to, time and again, remind yourself that the system was the first major attempt to explain the human condition from a yogic perspective. By examining the way the mind works, impermanence, and the nature of reality and perception itself, Sāṁkhya laid a remarkable groundwork for future thinkers to build on. Even though it had its limitations, and in spite of the fact that the system was often highly criticized by others, it presented ideas that have been instrumental in the development of both the yogic and Buddhist perspective. But because Sāṁkhya attempted to demonstrate the nature of mind and existence, there was (and still is) room for confusion on the part of those attempting to follow the subtle philosophical threads the system laid before us. This is due to the fact that we must use our own minds to understand the ideas about our own minds that Sāṁkhya presents. At first, conceptualizing puruṣa as something called pure consciousness and prakṛti as "all things that manifest" seems relatively simple and straightforward. However, because it is our mind, our "self," our own intimate connection to pure consciousness (but one filled with ego) that has the insight of understanding, and because that same mind is naturally and constantly producing more ideas—we are forever generating prakṛti—it is very easy for the concepts of Sāṁkhya to slip through our fingers as its ideas dissolve and fold back in on themselves. It can be confounding! But still it is worth returning to for a foundation in understanding.

Within a metaphorical representation, the Sāṁkhya world can be represented as a vehicle or chariot that the puruṣa rides around in. Eventually the gross aspect of the vehicle, our body, falls apart and dies, and the subtle information-holding aspect, a subtle body of buddhi—ahaṁkāra, manas, and subtle senses—then transmigrates to another vehicle until that body too dies. Another popular analogy represents prakṛti visually as a circular flower or maṇḍala. In such graphic representation, the puruṣa sits at the very center and experiences through the buddhi and prāṇa the various petal-like layers of the buddhi, ego function, and mind, which form our transmigrating subtle body. The next layer of the flower is the physical body and senses. These petals, located nearer the rim, interface with the petals of the outer world and with other beings, which form the outermost rim of petals. Each of us sits within our own slightly unique prakṛti maṇḍala or flower. Each flower is the whole world and therefore is both uniquely individualized while at the same time containing all of the other flowers. Remember that our individual subtle mind and gross body experience is represented as the more inner circles or our maṇḍala. The center of our own maṇḍala is in the heart, where riding on pillows of prāṇa (breath) or buddhi (intelligence) sits the puruṣa. When the heart is polished through deep meditation and devotion it becomes like a pristine mirror, reflecting the clear light of pure consciousness.

The flowerlike maṇḍala of prakṛti is in a constant state of change, folding back on itself, unfurling, and then refolding again and again. Petal by petal, layer by layer, the pattern folds back into its source so that it completely hugs the core, and then we open the pattern back up again. This, in fact, is how the process of yoga can work; the more layering and folding we do, the more deeply we are able to dissolve into and benefit from the effects of the yoga. The innermost shells of our prakṛti vehicle are the subtle body, where the most cherished aspirations, deep emotions, and commitments are, and where any control or choice from the ego principle might originate. Inside of this innermost circle of our maṇḍala is placed a dot, a bindu, which literally means "droplet." From this bindu, this point, time and space are said to unfold and then to enfold again and again. In the unfolding of time and space, buddhi, ahaṁkāra, and manas are revealed, and it is from this unfolding of these three aspects of mind that we experience the universe. Within the physical flowerlike maṇḍala of the body and senses, we may even experience pulsations that expand outward from the bindu followed reflexively by a response back in toward it. These pulsations, out of and back into our deepest core, pass through the subtle body, which both colors the pulsations and is also changed by them.

The bindu is surrounded by shells of deep emotion, feelings,

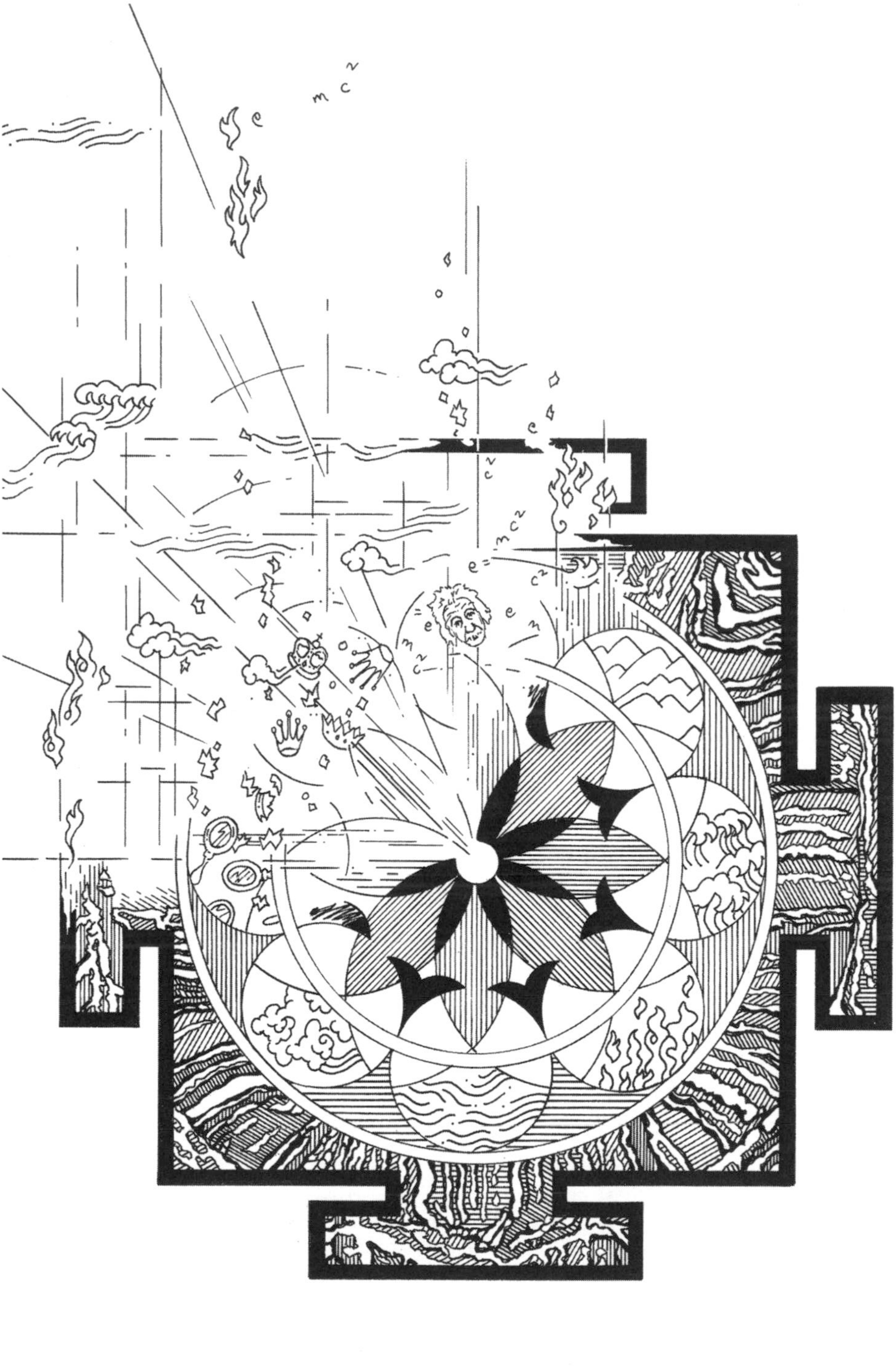
e=mc²

aspirations, dreams, and memories. Along with the bindu experience, these shells normally remain hidden below the level of our awareness. The outer accessible shell is the everyday awakened awareness, the screen of our consciousness. Thoughts, sensations, and forms make their loops through this screen of awareness, arising from unperceived depths of the mind and then returning to those same hidden roots of the unconscious mind. This system is dynamic: the conscious mind—the surface—moves or responds in a way that will affect the hidden core; the core in turn throws up new material onto the surface of awareness. In a dull, semi-awake mind, the response of the conscious mind is to accept or reject content based on the ego structure. This reaction to the content merely adds on to the growth pattern of the unconscious conditioning. When the intelligence begins to wake up, the conscious mind becomes sensitive to the dynamic interplay with the unconscious mind; first as awareness of feedback from the body, mind, and the environment; and later as a pulsation, or perhaps even as a dance of mindfulness with what is unmanifest or out of sight. The greater portion of the mind and the world must and will remain out of sight or hidden. There is a cryptic saying from the Upaniṣads: "The gods love what is out of sight."

With training in yoga, there is no fear of the hidden and no need for certainty. The buddhi stimulates continuous awakening with a limitless freedom to reframe experience by discovering links between the

Maṇḍala of Prakṛti (5)

This representation of the maṇḍala of prakṛti shows that all of its structures eventually break apart and dissolve back into undifferentiated energy. The maṇḍala represents our entire experience, both internally and externally, of the world and the mind. The gross external elements, their mental representations, the thoughts and ideas we have about them, our body and the gross or subtle bodies of even the highest and most subtle beings, are all part of this interconnected maṇḍala of creative energy. The pattern in the outer courtyard of the maṇḍala is that of a tortoiseshell. Traditionally the tortoise represents the underlying paradox of a support for all creation. Does the tortoise have another tortoise under it, or is it floating in empty, open sky?

focus and the horizon (the manifest and unmanifest). This underlying intelligence—the context maker—not only allows linkings that define and redefine relationship, but it also allows us to wake up or to move away from one context and into another. With intelligence turned toward puruṣa, there is the ability for an ever-deepening understanding of all perceptions so that the whole system becomes open and free. When the buddhi does not function well, it serves the false ego and is splayed out by the appearance of separate sense objects and conflicting needs. In this case our prakṛtic flower is simply a dream machine in which there is no awakening from the different fantasies of the mind and no ability to actually ascertain reality. The most important aspect of prakṛti, therefore, is the buddhi. In fact, all that we actually experience—the immediate surface of all internal or external sensation as well as thoughts, theories, and intuition that more exists behind the surface of our experience—is buddhi.

Buddhi is like an enchanted mirror. When ignorance prevails, the mirror presents the phantoms of endless forms and stories. The puruṣa identifies with those as in a bad dream. When the deepest talent of the buddhi is switched on, when we have discriminating awareness, which is called viveka khyātiḥ, then forms in the mirror are seen as interdependent with their entire background: they are seen as being empty of self, empty of puruṣa. Through the process of discriminating awareness we appreciate that we are always in intimate contact with buddhi, with the innermost and softest layer of the flower of prakṛti. This appreciation points out to us that ultimately the essential nature of our experience of prakṛti is simply the very nature of puruṣa, or of open pure consciousness.

Prakṛti is ultimately an empty mirror, reflecting the light of puruṣa. Or we could say prakṛti is the light shining through the open, empty nature of puruṣa. At this point we no longer have any image or metaphor for puruṣa, for pure consciousness. Puruṣa is not a thing, not a separate man or woman, nor an impulse, magnetism, or quality of any sort. Philosophically the concept of puruṣa has functioned as a meditation tool to keep the prakṛti open. Since puruṣa always slips out of any category of definition and is not a "thing" that can oppose prakṛti, the question arises as to whether the Sāṁkhya system is really a dualist system. Many schools of philosophical thought that came along after Sāṁkhya have asked the question, if puruṣa and prakṛti are completely separate, how then can they influence each other? And if everything that is perceived and thought is actually prakṛti, how do you even know or think about a puruṣa? Within the Sāṁkhya system all events and all phenomena, no matter what they are, are interrelated. This is so because *everything* within the Sāṁkhya system is part of the braiding of the guṇas of prakṛti and is open and empty of separate self. Consequently, when we describe the nature of prakṛti as complete openness, we end up describing puruṣa. It is enough to make the head spin! It is why Sāṁkhya philosophy is so difficult to stick with, so easily criticized, and it is also why Sāṁkhya is rejected by those who try to hold onto its meaning too literally and attempt to make the puruṣa into a thing, a symbol, a personification, or a form.

The problem with dualism is that it creates an unbridgeable gap between spirit and the world or, on a lower level, between the body and the mind. The gap is useful in order to understand concepts, but if we become too strict and unyielding in our thinking, we begin looking at the world as useless, miserable, impermanent, and bad. More often we even see the body as bad. Prejudged so, body and world are not really worthy of or interesting enough for our deep contemplation and appreciation, and we abandon our digging into the well of understanding Sāṁkhya.

It is said that the function of prakṛti is to reveal puruṣa, just as a mirror reveals whoever is gazing into it as themselves. It is also said that out of this mirroring of puruṣa through prakṛti, complete release or pure consciousness naturally radiates. At the end of the *Sāṁkhya Kārikā*, which is the main text on Sāṁkhya philosophy, there is a beautiful verse in which the puruṣa reveals that there is nothing more wonderful than prakṛti when she has been seen. This establishes a metaphor in which prakṛti is imagined to be an exquisite female dancer, moving gracefully, with absolutely no self-awareness at all, and puruṣa is the passive male observer. When prakṛti notices that she is being observed as herself, she becomes shy, which is actually her essential nature, and she ceases to dance, which causes her to unmanifest, at which point the flower of prakṛti is said to become smooth like the surface of a mirror. When prakṛti stops dancing in response to being seen, puruṣa is liberated and simply rests in his own true nature. This metaphor is to exemplify the process of yoga as one of simply watching things as they arise. We watch with a completely open mind, with undivided attention, awe and appreciation. The *Sāṁkhya Kārikā* explains:

> As a dancing girl ceases to dance having exhibited herself to an audience, so prakṛti ceases to manifest having exhibiting herself to puruṣa. . . . My opinion is that nothing is more modest than prakṛti: knowing that "I have been seen," she no longer comes within the sight of puruṣa. Thus, puruṣa is never bound, nor is he released nor does he transmigrate. Prakṛti, the support of the manifold creation, transmigrates, is bound and is released. . . . Thus from the practice of discriminating awareness is produced the wisdom: "I am not," "nothing is mine" and "not I," which is complete without residue, pure, and absolute. (Verses 59, 61, 62, and 64)

The puruṣa is empty of self, so the puruṣa is not a puruṣa (even though to conceptualize it, it had to be seen for just a moment as *a* thing). This paradox is good news. The dualism of Sāṁkhya is reconciled with the nondualism of the Upaniṣads. With continuous discriminating awareness there is no need to jump to conclusions about what we are observing and no need to look for or make an image of the puruṣa. In fact, now we can even witness the very thought that there is a "we" observing as "we" dissolve into the heart of the situation. If the mind begins to close and we start to draw conclusions about whatever we are watching, instantly that which is being observed becomes shy, and the true nature of the object we are observing disappears from view. Instead it transforms into a reflection of our direct experience in the mirror of our own mind.

Genuine deep yogic states, therefore, are those in which something appears in an unobstructed form. It is extraordinarily difficult for any of us to be able to maintain an unobstructed awareness of any experience because when an observation first registers, our own mind covers it, and the true unobstructed nature of that which is being observed instantly disappears. However, as we deepen our yoga practice, we find moments in which our instinct to understand, label, define, categorize, and judge that which we are witnessing can be suspended so that we simply see what we are seeing. This intensity of openness and awareness, the need for consistently refolding our awareness back on itself as we continuously reawaken our senses, summarizes the entire process of yoga.

As we have seen, an understanding of the system of Sāṁkhya can be elusive. The mind grasps it, then you blink and instantly the mind slips back into confusing puruṣa with prakṛti, forgetting the interlacing and supportive quality of the guṇas and the vital importance of buddhi and manas. It can be helpful once again to imagine the system as a geometric diagram, shaped like a flower with petals folded closed toward the center. If you take the center of that diagram and pull upward on it, as if you were pulling open a vegetable-steaming basket or the flower itself, it will unfold and will start to form the cakra system as used in the internal visualizations of the haṭha and the tantric yoga traditions. Another useful way to imagine a use for the Sāṁkhya system is to place a hole in the center of our flower or maṇḍala image. This way there is no "thing" in its very center, and you begin to understand that the wheel of Sāṁkhya is actually empty, that at its core is space. Looking at Sāṁkhya in this way you can easily draw a parallel to the Buddhist perspective in which all of the components, all of the elements of the universe, are in their deep essence empty of self.

The influence of other schools and mythologies has made the puruṣa-prakṛti model personable and easier to understand. Since nondualism ultimately considers the world itself to be the ātman (the Self), prakṛti was no longer represented as unconscious, purely mechanical, dead energy. She became a vibrant goddess, and puruṣa is discovered to be the lover of this goddess. They are not two: each is without self and has as its essence, as its heart, the other. They are not one: their interplay generates joy and constant discovery of the moment of their linking together. This apparent upgrading of the Sāṁkhya philosophy directly demonstrates how the mythologies of Rādhā and Kṛṣṇa, of Sītā and Rāma, of Śiva and Śakti are easily formulated. Each of these famous pairs of divinities within Indian mythology are in the most intimate relationship with each other; in the heart of Kṛṣṇa rests his beloved, Rādhā, and in Rādhā's heart is her true love, Kṛṣṇa, and so it is too with Sītā and Rāma, Śiva and Śakti. This interdependent relationship allows us to experience the world on all levels inside and out as a combining and recombining of these two, who are like the two ends of a stick, not really two. This can be experienced immediately as the interdependent wave of prāṇa and apāna in our yoga practice. The two play together, they interpenetrate and occasionally come into suspension or union. This working metaphor of deep interconnectedness expands our understanding of our core emotions, allowing us to really grasp the richness of our being through relationship with the other.

In this light we can see the Sāṁkhya universe to be beyond but not opposed to historical views of the world. The beginning of time is defined as the present moment, not some 13.7 billion years ago at the time of the big bang. The beginning of the universe is right now, right here in the present moment. Our universe, from a Sāṁkhya perspective, is simultaneously being given to us just as it is being created by us. It is constantly expanding out from the present moment and then returning back into the present, moment by moment. What is even more remarkable about the Sāṁkhya universe is that you can actually experience this perspective through your own body; it is not simply a theoretical model of the universe to be understood cognitively through study. Instead it is an understanding of the direct, vibrant, pulsating nature of the creative energy that we are always immersed in. All of the different practices of yoga, therefore, bring the universe of prakṛti to life as direct and immediate experiences rather than as simple descriptions that are to be written in notebooks and memorized.

We find, therefore, that the study of yoga might include examining the history of different schools of yoga. It might also involve studying different philosophies and contemplations about yoga that the seers have made over thousands of years of practice. But primarily in yoga we are studying our own immediate experience, and the Sāṁkhya system is like a road map that helps you observe your own experience very closely. In that sense the Sāṁkhya universe begins now with your own circumstances, with the present sensations and feelings and thoughts you are experiencing, just as they are. But the universe also ends right now by fully and openly—without an overlay of theory and preconception—observing those very same things.

6

The *Bhagavad Gītā* and the Unfolding of Love

I bow to the Madhava, the supreme bliss, by whose grace the lame can cross mountains and the dumb can speak eloquently.

—The *Gītā Dhyānam*, verse 8, a collection of eight verses that glorify the *Bhagavad Gītā*

All of the different schools and philosophies of yoga are rooted in a composite of traditions that stretch back beyond five thousand years. In ancient times teachers would have periods of formal teaching followed by an intermission. During these breaks either they or another teacher would tell stories that exemplified the teachings in order to pass the essence of their message along in a fashion that more people would understand. Those listening to the storytelling could relate the tales to their own experience, to their feelings, and their lives, which allowed them to intuit the meaning and to grapple with life's deeper significance and underlying philosophical paradoxes. Eventually these stories and myths were bundled together into longer narratives that meander through the different attitudes, viewpoints, and methods that comprise most of the different schools of yoga. Classical myths from all cultures function as metaphors for life, and some are even layers upon layers of metaphors. They serve to awaken awareness deep inside the core of your being by stimulating certain emotions, experiences, and archetypes that may be forgotten or overlooked during daily life. Given this metaphorical format, it is important not to take mythology too literally, but it is equally important to allow the insight inspired by the stories to be absorbed. Soaking up the message from mythology is like learning from a good theater production—you must buy into the story, believe the characters and problems to be real, and emotionally ride on the action of the story line in order for it to work. In the West we are familiar with the stories of the *Iliad* and the *Odyssey*, the mythological epics that grew out of a storytelling tradition in ancient Greece. These epic tales were part of people's daily lives long before the great philosophical schools arose within the Greek culture. In a similar fashion the *Mahābhārata* grew to be the great Indian epic, told again and again over generations. *Mahā* means "greater" or "extended." *Bharata* means the "greater land of the ancient king Bharat" (in fact, India today is called Bharata). The *Mahābhārata*, therefore, is an expansive collection of stories relating to the ancient kingdoms of India. The *Mahābhārata* is not one myth but instead a compilation of myths that fit together; they are woven so intricately as one that it becomes almost impossible to step back and identify any particular part of the myth as the final frame of the story. It goes on, merging subplots into the main plot, circling out to new narrators and back to old ones. It is interesting to imagine an even bigger version of the *Mahābhārata* as the story of everything, in which we might even find the stories of our own lives—those same plots and subplots that go around and around in our own minds. Next time you notice your mind creating a proposition, a narrative, or a story line, know that from this point of view, your self-image is simply a character in a subchapter of the extended version of the *Mahābhārata*!

One of the greatest texts for studying the variety of schools of yoga is the *Bhagavad Gītā*, "The Song of God," which is part of the *Mahābhārata*. It is the climax of the story of Prince Arjuna, the warrior who finds himself in a moral and spiritual crisis, confused about what action to take under dire circumstances. The book opens on the famous battlefield called the Kurukṣetra where opposing armies have gathered after a long struggle between two political dynasties, one good and one evil. On one side of the battlefield are Arjuna and Yudhiṣṭhira, his elder brother and the rightful king. With them are Arjuna's younger brothers and his fellow warriors, all of noble and good character. On the other side of the battlefield are their cousins, all considered to be troublemakers, and who are led by Duryodhana, the evil son of the blind and weak King Dhṛtarāṣṭra who is the usurper of the kingdom. Arjuna's crisis is that although he understands the events leading up to the battle and feels deep alignment with the warriors on his side, upon looking across the field at the faces of his opponents, he sees many of his cousins, friends, and teachers. He is overwhelmed and immobilized by conflict, knowing that whatever action he takes, people he cares deeply about will be harmed. Neither of the sides is totally bad nor is either side totally good. Arjuna becomes caught in a dilemma in which he understands that no matter what action he takes, the consequences of his actions and the problems that may arise as a result are bound to be horrible. Perhaps no more difficult a situation could have been presented to Arjuna. The root of the crisis is that Arjuna is a very good person with a sweet and open heart; he is kind, compassionate, and extremely honest. He finds himself in a truly human situation in which he feels his own conflict and sense of anguish, but he also perceives the incredible amount of suffering that is going on around him. Arjuna realizes that all of the formulas and religious systems that he has studied and immersed himself in—all of his theories and techniques—will not salvage the situation, and that no matter what he does, his actions or nonactions will result in many deaths and the possible destruction of the culture he truly loves.

Arjuna's teacher, who is the god Kṛṣṇa, happens also to be his charioteer in the battle. In Indian mythology Kṛṣṇa represents the archetype of the guru and is considered to be the teacher of teachers, the innermost self in the heart of all beings, and the Bhagavad Gītā is carefully crafted to point out to the astute reader (the listener) the parallel between themselves and Arjuna. Kṛṣṇa informs Arjuna that he is lost in a world of name and form and that his body is merely a very brief phenomenon within a tapestry of change. Arjuna's initial response to confronting the temporary nature of all things is one of immense depression and fear. Just as he realizes that he is already in the process of dying, so too in following the story the intelligent reader also recognizes the nature of impermanence in all things and sees that they themselves are presently in the process of dying; that the temporary nature of all things is a fact of life.

The *Bhagavad Gītā* is so skillfully crafted that carefully reading it allows you to appreciate the fact of impermanence not only intellectually, but by actually feeling it in your skin and by experiencing its meaning in your muscles and bones. Perhaps this is one reason the book has had such a long and lasting effect, because through such a visceral understanding there is an opportunity for profound insight into the nature of reality. When you experience the vibration of your breath and you truly recognize the vibratory quality of everything you encounter, when you feel constant change in all that is going on around you right now, then you have deep insight into the meaning of life. However, when first presented with this all-encompassing nature of impermanence you may, as Arjuna did, become depressed and filled with fear and doubt. If you pay close attention to this very state of mind as it arises within you, you might notice your breath has quickened, which is an excellent indicator of your own vulnerability—of your heart opening to the reality of your own impermanence—which it turns out is the only way to navigate the situation with compassion and intelligence.

Anyone who has ever been in a relationship with another person knows that as you open the gates of your heart a taste of this crisis—the predicament of dying—always arises. This is because if you are truly going to experience another person as they actually are, rather than projecting your theories, preconceptions, or mind states onto them, you must surrender or at least suspend those theories. To be in an ongoing relationship, whether it is with a friend, a lover, a teacher, or simply a casual acquaintance, you must step out of the way. Stuck in a world of name and form Arjuna was at the point where he needed to give up not only his concepts and images of himself, but more important, he needed to give up concepts and images of the other warriors and people in his life. From there he could then relinquish his fixed ideas about society, religion, and dharma. A profound and not always obvious facet of the teaching in the opening of the *Gītā* therefore is the universal nature of impermanence that we share with all embodied beings and with all forms and manifestations. This insight of all-pervasive impermanence was the precondition for Arjuna's enlightenment just as it is for any of us; we must be open and attentive both inwardly and outwardly.

The very first verse of the *Bhagavad Gītā* reads, "Here, in the field of dharma [dharma kṣetra], here in the field of action [Kuru kṣetra], assembled together, eager to fight, what did my army and the army of the Pandavas do?" (Pandavas is the name of Arjuna's family.) The word *kṣetra* means "field," *dharma* means "duty, truth, religion, law, and the fundamental constituents of all things," and *kuru* means "action." So the story begins where the fields of dharma, religion, and deep idealism meet the field of action in practical, grounded necessity. When you find yourself in any situation in which your circumstances require you to do something, you must act, and your actions must be in accordance with your own sense of truth within your circumstances. The entire story of the *Bhagavad Gītā* is a playing out of what happens inside each of us whenever we unroll our mat to do our yoga practice. It is as if we are stepping onto the field of dharma and the field of kuru as we draw together the deep truths represented in the yoga practice and take some form of action within the practice to connect to the unique particulars of the body and mind at that moment. We are compelled by whatever reason to come to the mat and to begin a practice. Exactly what has brought us to yoga, precisely what our intentions are in terms of the practice, and what we actually do once we are on the mat are variables that are completely different person to person and often day to day for any one of us. "Should I try hard, and express the radiance and joy of the ātman, or should I take it easy, and remain sleepy, dull, and safe? Should I push to extremes, and injure myself, or should I take a step back and just bask in the sunshine?" Questions like these go on and on in different forms and combinations every time we practice. The answers to our inquisitiveness are not always obvious. As we step onto the mat, we are stepping into the middle of a battlefield between two armies of choices and counterchoices, of thoughts and counterthoughts so that we may deal with the particularity and the totality of our circumstances. Like Arjuna, we might find we need a little advice.

The hero of the *Bhagavad Gītā*, the prince Arjuna, deeply enmeshed in an unpleasant fratricidal war, is caught in a spiritual and practical dilemma. Neither side is totally good nor totally bad; the two sides are interdependent like the sides of a coin. Neither the arguments for fighting nor the lines of reasoning against the battle are airtight. If he decides not to do anything, then the evil army will conquer the good army. This would cause great anguish for the entire culture because the unjust rulers would take over, resulting in mayhem for the whole civilization. If, on the other hand, he decides *to* fight the so-called righteous war, then many and maybe all of the noble people on both sides would be killed. Ultimately even though the outcome of this choice of action would mean the establishment of a more just and conscious social order, it might not be worth it because many of those who could enjoy such a good kingdom would be dead. In the presence of his friend Kṛṣṇa, the archetype of the teacher or the guru, Arjuna sobers up to the situation and has his moment of full spiritual crisis. He calls a time-out, and it is during that pause that the telling of the story of the *Bhagavad Gītā* unfolds. Perhaps no more difficult situation could have been presented to Arjuna. It was tailored to trap him at a crossroads where formulas and habitual responses would not do. This dilemma is a brilliant representation of our very own human circumstance, where at critical times in life each of us finds ourselves within our own unique versions of Arjuna's crisis.

Part of the conflict that Arjuna feels is a result of his being already an advanced and intelligent yogin, a compassionate man with a job as a warrior that requires (when unavoidable) some violent action. His problem is that he lives in an imperfect society with rules that are flawed, so that no matter what action he might take, there is bound to be a great deal of suffering. A major theme in the *Bhagavad Gītā* is that all of our actions have some element of imperfection to them. The outcome of any given action might be good, but it will not be absolutely perfect. Even those actions that seem to be bad actions will most likely contain some good elements or will result in some positive effect. Likewise, all systems of practice (yogic, religious, political, and so on) have some imperfection to them; they all have some blind spot. So if you practice a system unwaveringly, something will remain unaddressed or unresolved, and there is likely to be residue from the practice and some aspect of your life that remains unconscious. Under these circumstances where action must be taken, we run into the familiar notion that you are damned if you do and damned if you don't; however, the *Bhagavad Gītā* offers the insight that the residue of work, when experienced with the same attentiveness given to our original dilemma of crisis, keeps us from falling back into reducing beings and things to just name and form. The story of the *Gītā* is a demonstration of how to stop the cycle of a crisis being resolved by a solution that just creates another crisis later. Acknowledging the nature of names, forms, theories, and techniques as being incomplete, the *Gītā* opens the door to love, and it is from here that the tale unfolds.

The first formal teaching that the smiling Kṛṣṇa offers to the dejected Arjuna is the underlying principle of Sāṁkhya yoga. He explains to Arjuna the notion that there never was a time when he or Arjuna (or all of the warriors on the field or any being, for that matter) did not exist, nor will there ever be a time when they will cease to be. He explains that just as we pass from childhood through youth and old age, so at death we take another body and that the wise are not confused by this. Kṛṣṇa illuminates the idea that the bodies of all the warriors on the battlefield are going to die, because they are compositions of the creative energy, prakṛti (which by nature is always changing). The bodies of those warriors, like the bodies of all living creatures, are impermanent. Even if the warriors survive this battle, they are eventually all going to die. He continues to make clear that from this perspective what really counts is the ātman, the puruṣa, the true self. This ātman, which is both all-pervading and localized in each of us, is indestructible and changeless. Even though the body changes and dies, the ātman does not. With this insight, Arjuna sees that in order to resolve his crisis, he needs to follow the path of buddhi yoga, or the yoga of insightful intelligence. A clean and integrated buddhi leads to discriminative knowledge, or the ability to discriminate between that which is the permanent and whole and that which is illusory and impermanent. *Buddhi yoga* is the term used in Sāṁkhya to refer to a broader approach called jñāna yoga, that of knowledge or wisdom. Arjuna learns that simply understanding the value of discriminative knowledge is not enough, that the insight must be integrated into a broad and complete understanding of the human condition in order for it to be truly insightful.

Through the continuation of the story of the *Bhagavad Gītā*, it is shown that although it may be true that the ability to discriminate is imperative, it is also important to recognize that even the most powerful insight into the nature of reality is itself reflected in ideas that are part of prakṛti. The structures and containers of the insight must eventually be released. With wisdom alone the intelligence tends to create a subtle ego or knower hidden in the background. This can result in a sense of pride and might create a disdain for the world and for the ignorant. Even the wisdom contained within jñāna yoga itself, however, must dissolve back into the heart rather than turning into a dogma, because then it will be the theory rather than the truth of the ideas that drives action and thought. For example, if you go up to a stranger on the street and begin to explain to them that everything is an illusion, and then proceed to attempt an explanation of the entire Sāṁkhya system of yoga, you will probably get a look of great confusion or disbelief. Someone not immersed in an in-depth philosophical inquiry into the meaning of life is likely to think you are presenting a very depressing view of reality—that everything is an illusion and that it is temporary to boot—even though that philosophical standpoint might be cosmologically true. This is part of the problem philosophers run into; when Sāṁkhya yoga (or any perspective for that matter) is presented as dry and dogmatic, it completely misses out on the root of philosophy—which is an attempt to explain and get back to the ecstasy and richness of the human experience, shedding light on what is going on deep in the core of our hearts as dharmas meet the real world of practical action.

Within the story of the *Bhagavad Gītā*, Arjuna is the perfect character to receive and filter an understanding of the teachings because his heart is so open and so sensitive that he has the innate capacity to allow his insights to dissolve back again and again into his own heart and through his own buddhi. For instance, when he finds himself on the battlefield, he feels compassion for all participants on both sides in the impending battle. Before the fighting is to begin, he is so deeply moved that his mouth feels parched and his hair stands on end. He feels weak and his bow drops from his hand as he is swept by an overwhelming wave of compassion and of not-knowing what action to take. Kṛṣṇa's initial teaching of Sāṁkhya yoga leaves Arjuna even more confused and thoroughly perplexed. So Kṛṣṇa then proceeded to teach Arjuna karma yoga, which has a much more inviting and human face to it.

Karma yoga is the yoga of doing something; it is the yoga of work. As we all know, one of the best therapies in life is to just go out and work, to get your hands into something. Good old work will get you off of your high horse of theories and bring you down to earth because you have to use and abandon techniques and tools as you adapt and readapt to real situations. The beginning of karma yoga is the need to eat, to survive, and perhaps to get a paycheck. The result of that food or paycheck is the survival and hopefully the health of body and family. Body and family are not the happiness, joy, or the final goal or purpose of work: wisdom and compassion are. The underlying premise of karma yoga is that as you work, you should work eventually for the joy of working rather than becoming attached to the fruits of your labors. If you work to become wealthy or to become famous, if you work with the motivation of doing a good deed, or of becoming a better person, you can easily become attached to those goals and those ideas of who you are, and you can also become attached to the fruits of your work. Perhaps, for example, you have done so many good deeds that others frequently tell you how important your work is and how valuable you are—things just wouldn't be the same without you. Soon you begin to consider yourself quite generous and magnanimous, and before long it is difficult for you to imagine how the world could get along without you; you have become enamored with and attached to the image you have of yourself as the openhearted and talented person that your work has shown you to be. This is a natural progression of the function of mind—especially when others bolster your ego with compliments—and it provides an opportunity to either bite the bait and fall into a realm of self-absorption or to step back and observe the workings of your mind rejecting it or holding on tightly.

The distinguishing feature of karma yoga is that even though you may offer the fruits of your work to the benefit of others, you honestly do not have any expectations whatsoever that you will gain anything from that offering. In this way work itself is important to you, and eventually the work becomes art. In the yogic sense of the word, art is more than creating a pretty design, an accurate replica of something in life, or a fine representation of some aspect of religion. Instead it is a connection through the heart to the very essence of one's being—a connection to the truth within everyone's being. In this light, the quintessence of the path of karma yoga is the understanding that yoga is the *art* of work. Such non-self-conscious art is naturally beneficial to others.

As we undertake any task, begin any work, we find ourselves embarking on a process that can eventually lead us to insight and to truth, even though in the beginning we may be a little bit confused by a situation that seems to be presenting many different ideas and options for action. This is the same confusion Arjuna experienced when faced with the dilemma of which action to take, and it happens any time we are presented with multiple choices between which we must choose in order to act. But because in order to work we are obliged to take some action, we gradually begin to gain knowledge about the situation and the impact of our work, which makes us better at the work when we return to it the next time. If we stick with the essence of the work itself, rather than focusing on the fruits of our actions, we eventually find ourselves in the presence of truth. This is how karma yoga works—we simply begin by taking conscious action, working with great care, then naturally the quality of our work is integrated into the context of the situation and the work is therefore excellent. Because we work with no expectations and no attachment to the payback, the outcome in terms of what we are going to get out of the work, we can then work with deep concentration, an open mind, and an open heart. This is actually how people become incredibly efficient at their work and extraordinarily gifted in the art or their actions. If you have ever studied a musical instrument you may have experienced this process. Until the music is so very smooth and seamless, until you can play as if there is nobody performing, but in a manner that the music simply flows on its own, then there is tension in your body and distraction in your mind. When learning an instrument you eventually find yourself at a point where you have failed so many times that you have finally given up any attachment to the by-product of your performance, and it is only *then* that you can melt into the music and finally start playing the instrument simply for the sake of playing it. This is the underlying feeling inspired through karma yoga. There is always a great aesthetic pleasure that results from this kind of work, and it is through the aesthetic experience that we then discover our deep connection with other beings. Karma yoga may appear as our desire to help others or to serve others, whether they are immediate family or friends, or whether our actions come as a desire to serve society as a whole. When we are doing work that really needs to be done in such a way that the work itself becomes joyous, then we are doing karma yoga. You must be willing to really get your hands in there and engage with whatever form the work takes when doing karma yoga. Even if it is the most simple or menial type of work, the work itself becomes an essential path, and in this way all other types of yoga become supported by the activity of karma yoga. In fact no matter what type of yoga practice you take up, you will find that karma yoga is an operating and crucial element within it. Through karma yoga the work itself becomes an experience of aesthetics and beauty—the *experience* of art that inspires a depth of appreciation for the grounding and visceral nature of the aesthetic experience. Because it is so fulfilling to work in this way, when your aesthetic sense is gratified, it is quite simple to develop a healthy detachment from the fruits of your actions. In fact, this is the same detachment that Kṛṣṇa was hoping Arjuna would experience as he gained the insight that his ability to work with detachment rested in an understanding of Sāṁkhya philosophy.

The story of the *Bhagavad Gītā* demonstrates the necessity of certain types of work (in Arjuna's case, the necessity of participating in the battle), and it also demonstrates that through an understanding of work as an aesthetic experience, a significant concept of dharma becomes clear. One of the many important meanings of dharma is as your own true, deep individual nature. Looking at dharma in this light, we see that there are different types of things that you must do in order to fulfill yourself. These things are closely associated with the real necessities that are part of the circumstances of your own life, and they, too, are considered to be your dharma. For some of us, for example, it turns out that our dharma is the necessity of getting a job and learning to deal with financial matters. For others it is the necessity that we create art or that we compose music. Or sometimes our dharma might be that we give up painting or composing in order to care for our ailing parents. All of these different and unique sets of circumstances are our individual dharmas, which define the genuine work that is laid out for us. It is vital to realize that we need to do what we truly have to do for ourselves in relation to our unique historical circumstances. Who and where we are in relation to the rest of our lives—our family, our past choices and actions, the state of the world—all of these things help to determine the dharmic path we pursue. It is also very important to remember, as is pointed out in the *Bhagavad Gītā*, that it is better to do your own dharma poorly than to do someone else's dharma well. In other words, it is essential that each of us follow our own individual dharma. Rather than pursuing your own conveniently imagined dharma, oblivious of its effect on others, and rather than taking on the dharma of someone else and in so doing avoiding the work and relationships that really connect deep into your own heart and gut, your actual dharma must be in tune with the truth within you in the context of your actual circumstances.

Often when we engage in an activity or some work, we discover that there is some small imperfection to our image of what that work is. We develop a great idea, a great plan, but when we actually execute it we discover the occasional rough edge, or we run into some by-product that we had not anticipated. Kṛṣṇa explains to Arjuna that just like fire always has smoke, so too whatever you do always has a residue of imperfection. Eventually either you have to offer the residue itself into the fire of your own consciousness, or you have to go back and create another little project to deal with that residue. This is why people who are perfectionists seem always to be working: they are constantly going back to tidy up the edges as nothing is ever explained perfectly nor is anything ever done correctly. This process of dealing with the residue can go on to infinity and is true even within our yoga practice. If you are a relentless perfectionist you will occasionally, almost by accident, come to the point of being absorbed by the pure art of the practice; we find these points when, perhaps unintentionally, we have offered our practice—our work and its residue—back into its source. It is when you give up perfectionism that you are able to appreciate a sense of fullness or completeness in a yoga pose. If this intention of offering the practice back into its source is not part of the practice, then the yoga practice itself can become the best system of self-torture ever devised; perfectionists love to grab it and misuse it that way. Remember dharma is specific to the individual; if you are not a perfectionist, then giving up perfectionism is not the best path.

A superficial inadequacy of the karma yoga system, if taken alone, is that we easily fall into the mind-set that yoga is something mechanical, that if we simply perform certain specific actions, we will get certain specific results. There is actually a whole school of Indian philosophy, called Karma Mīmāṁsā, which is a school composed of precise ritual. The underlying philosophy of this school is that if you simply perform a series of extraordinarily detailed rituals without mistake, then you are certain to get the benefit of the ritual—which is essentially that you go straight to heaven. The theory within this school is that the gods will grant you certain rewards if you mechanically follow specific rules. Of course the fallacy in this thinking is that it reduces the universe to merely a machine, and in so doing it reduces the principle of relationship with others to a predetermined mechanical prison. Another inadequacy of karma yoga taken alone is that when work does become art, it does not really provide the language or the refinement of methodology to deal with the deep aesthetic experience that is stimulated through the execution of the work. So in the story of the *Bhagavad Gītā*, after teaching Arjuna about karma yoga, Kṛṣṇa introduces the practice of sacrifice called yajña.

All action and all work are ultimately an investment of energy and time that produce some form of result. To not be attached to that result, to give up the fruit of your actions, is the art of karma. Sacrifice or yajña brings into that act of giving up the intention of offering the results—the whole process—to another. This expands our view of everything we have and all that we do into a greater matrix beyond our own self-centered needs. In the ancient Vedic religion, sacrifices were made to the various gods as a gesture to please and nourish the gods as a means of lubricating the cycles of nature. In turn, the gods would make the rains fall on time, so that the crops would grow; crops could then be harvested and eaten as sacrifice; and many offerings to the gods could be made so that the whole wheel of the good life would continue. Even if you do not believe in a poly- or a pantheistic cosmos, an understanding of this interpenetrating nature of all things can still make sense if you consider the gods to represent the deeper patterns and collections of ideas in the buddhi. Through yoga sacrifice can be experienced viscerally, by observing how the actions you offer as sacrifice have a profound effect on your own deep mind, emotions, and the current functioning of the ego, the ahaṁkāra. What we could call our inner gods are functions of the ideas we have about who we and others are. Appearing as forces and impulses beyond our control, they are how we give value to things, how we rate the results of actions, and how we image our intentions and plans. In the Vedic age the principle ritual of offering to both inner and outer gods was the fire sacrifice, in which various symbolic items were poured or placed into the fire. The vision ultimately revealed by these practices of yajña was that all of the things and processes of our life are interdependent and that they move in cycles of renewal that are kept in motion through the act of sacrifice.

In the *Bhagavad Gītā*, Kṛṣṇa introduces a refined interpretation of the ancient religious sacrifice. Kṛṣṇa says that he himself, as the ātman (the Self) within the heart of all beings, is the true receiver of sacrifice. Being the ātman of all of the gods too, he has no ulterior motives nor does he desire the fruit of anyone's actions. He is not bound by work in any way. With this in mind as we ourselves practice the art of work as sacrifice, we can experience a sense of freedom and can become unbound by our own work in the same way. The immense satisfaction arising from this form of practice allows us to understand one of the core mysteries of the *Bhagavad Gītā;* we can see inaction in action, and action in inaction, the beautiful nondual vision of the world in which our bodies and minds are without a self. To truly understand this paradoxical action-inaction formula, we must peel back the layers through which it unfolds into its background. The first layer, revealed in the context of our understanding of Sāṁkhya, might be understood like this: when we experience either action or movement within the body or the mind, it is prakṛti acting on prakṛti. You (as puruṣa, the true you) are not doing anything. There are many ways of saying this same thing. Action done without attachment, without a sense of selfish interest, produces no karma or further attachment that must be resolved in the future. Such conscious work produces wisdom or jñāna. "Yoga is the art of action," says Kṛṣṇa. The following well-known verse of the *Gītā* sums up the mystery of the cycle of nature: "Brahman is the act of offering; Brahman is the oblation, poured by Brahman into the fire of Brahman. Brahman is attained by one who experiences that action and Brahman are one and the same" (IV. 24). Generally, our minds picture Brahman as the quiet substratum of pure, infinite joy, which exists beyond time. Forms, actions, and even vibrations are understood to be different. This is due to the natural way our minds make images and concepts of Brahman in order to be able think about what Brahman might mean. Ultimately, however, forms, actions and vibrations all interconnect without end, so ultimately they are not different from Brahman.

You can see a deep yoga practice as an internalized form of the classic Vedic fire sacrifice if you imagine pure awareness to be the fire. Within the *Bhagavad Gītā* we find suggestions for ways to actually experience this. For example, we can offer the sense objects, like sounds, smells, or any objectified sensation, into the fires of our senses. We can offer all of our sense actions and the actions of our prāṇa into the fire of pure consciousness. The prāṇa, which controls inhaling, can then be offered into the apāna, which controls exhaling, and we can then turn around and offer the apāna back into the prāṇa. (This, of course, is the basis of prāṇāyāma practice.) In fact, in the story of the *Gītā*, Kṛṣṇa mentions many, many variations of yogic sacrifice, almost as if to eliminate divisive and sectarian misunderstanding of the practice.

Finally Kṛṣṇa introduces the idea of knowledge as the ultimate sacrifice. Knowledge or jñāna is a product of action and conscious sacrifice. On a simple level consider the act of shooting an arrow from a new bow. The first shot lands short of the target, giving you information, and you adjust your aim. The second shot goes too far left, and you correct for that. Soon you and the bow are calibrated, and the art of archery is now carried in your mind and flesh as jñāna specific to archery, the new bow, and the circumstances at hand. With no action—with no shooting, missing, and correcting—there can be no real, grounded knowledge. Concentrated internal sacrifice, with its processes of gathering together materials of all levels of subtlety and then offering and letting them go in sacrifice, gradually increases our understanding of interconnectedness to the point of insight into the nature of all things. The sacrifice of knowledge is understood in two ways. First that the sacrifice—all work for that matter—is done with the understanding that work is selfless; it is a joy in and of itself and therefore produces no delusion or ignorance in oneself or in others. The second is that one must give up or sacrifice knowledge. Jñāna of course is not a thing that can be tossed in the fire, but the formulas, symbols, partial philosophies, and language games that are vehicles of pure intelligence burn beautifully. They must be seen through as context dependent structures, just like the gross, tangible objects all around us. Sacrificing them means entering into a state of not knowing, of having no image of self or other.

By the sixth chapter of the *Bhagavad Gītā*, Kṛṣṇa decides to teach Arjuna dhyāna yoga, the yoga of meditation. He introduces the formal structure of classical yoga practice as meditation. He carefully helps Arjuna to avoid many of the obstacles and misunderstandings that often arise within that austere path by placing it within a broad vision of integrated aesthetics, as part of the direct experience of the world of our everyday lives. Through this kind of focus of mind you can gain a direct experience of the heart—the ātman—which is simply pure consciousness. Even a fleeting encounter with the ātman reveals that there is nothing greater that could ever be experienced or attained; it is a completely satisfying experience. The taste of reality is so profound that even in the face of the most confusing dilemma or the greatest sorrow—even in the face of death—those who have experienced pure consciousness are not shaken from the deep internal experience of yoga. All yoga is aimed at this state of being, and in particular the practice of dhyāna yoga because it trains the mind, thought by thought, to be open to the experience of pure consciousness. Kṛṣṇa, by exposing Arjuna to yoga as meditation in this way, was giving him enough of a taste of reality that he could face with strength and clarity the situation before him on the battlefield.

Within the story of the *Bhagavad Gītā*, Kṛṣṇa is very careful to point out to Arjuna that yoga is not for someone who "lights no fire," meaning it is not for someone who experiences detachment due to laziness or avoidance of the rigor of work. Instead yoga is for those who are deeply inspired, who work in a focused, concentrated way while remaining truly nonattached to the fruits of their labor. Kṛṣṇa explains that when one is beginning the path of yoga, karma (work) is said to be the path. In this context, work may mean the actual activity of studying or of doing the yoga āsanas, or of carefully observing sensations and feelings within the body as they arise. There are phases of sitting meditation practice that are excruciating and can only be called hard work. We want easy pleasure, but the mind might be presenting sensation patterns, emotions, neurotic thought patterns, or hellish situations, which are reflexively rejected. We tend to jump away, thinking that meditation is not working or that we are failures or that we need a different teacher. Yet the simple requirement of mindfulness practice or discriminating awareness practice is to "sit with it" or to "see it just as it is." This is easy to say but not so easy to do when the shadow side of our ego rises up as the content of our consciousness. Seeing through concepts of pain and hell are absolutely vital to yoga practice. Otherwise we might think that we are advanced practitioners when in fact we suffer from ego inflation. The initial work of yoga, therefore, is to carefully observe your mind as you begin to stretch out the breath in prāṇāyāma, as you begin to engage the body in āsana, and as the whole spectrum of a mind-created heaven and hell unfold in actual meditation practice. By learning to stay attentive and focused within these aspects of yoga, you discover that the true work is the fervent, passionate inquiry into the present moment, into what is actually arising, as it arises. For the beginner therefore, work is the means to liberation.

For someone who has attained yoga and is actually awakened, *inaction* or ceasing action is said to be the means. In other words, once you are awakened to the nature of reality, when through an experience of pure consciousness you can be in the present moment, then you allow the universe to do its thing. All of the deep inner mechanisms of the mind and ego, of the senses and the prāṇa, all of these things will flow on their own once you have done the initial work required. At that point all you have to do is to continue to get out of the way. So if you are still a beginner in practice and the mind is held captive by conditioned experiences, conditioned thoughts, then your work is to observe those patterns of conditioning. When you have opened up the central channel of the body, and the blockage of the kuṇḍalinī at the lower opening of the central channel has been removed so that the prāṇa spontaneously enters the central path, *then* the practice is merely to relish the openness of the aesthetic experience. Beware: the ego structure is clever in its means of avoiding dissolution. Many yogins like to imagine that they are advanced to the point where inaction is their path. In actuality they lack the ability to focus the mind like a laser, to see through the games ego plays in their mind, and to be content and clear even as the dark shadow side of their fakery is exposed.

The classic systems of yoga are accompanied by all kinds of images that are traditionally associated with them. There is the image of the ascetic living in the mountains as a hermit, or of the meditator sitting for days and days on her deerskin, or of the yogi doing postures—sitting twisted up like a pretzel outside of his cave. Yet all of these associations leave something out because they are only descriptions of what is happening from an outside point of view rather than the internal experience of the yogi. The joy of yoga lies in finding your true self and the freedom that this affords. As you practice yoga you begin to realize that so many other beings, just like you, are still caught in the tangles and turnings of what is referred to as the wheel of saṁsāra, the wheel of conditioned existence. Then you begin to have insight into the fact that no matter how thorough the description, or how complete the methodology, no words and no theory can really express how to attain the freedom of yoga. The insight afforded through yoga is a completely unique and personal experience. Within the classical yoga systems, one of the key elements essential to attaining this form of enlightenment is that of surrender, which is often described as surrendering to God. Another method for attaining enlightenment is to simply drop the seed of your concentration, if you have such a seed, into not-knowing. Essentially these are the same thing because if you are to surrender, you must trust the nature of reality. You must give up your theories, techniques, and methods so that you can be free and present to simply *be* with whatever is appearing in the immediate experience of the moment at hand. The question, of course, is how to do that. In fact there is not really a specific formula that insures you will know how or be able to give up theories, techniques, or methods. The same is true, for example, if you are learning how to create art from a talented artist. The teacher can show you all sorts of methods and techniques, but she cannot really offer you a specific method or technique that insures you will become a great artist. Instead you must take the teachings and you must apply them; you must grapple with applying them to absorb their meaning and their application. To become a great artist yourself you must work at honing your skill so that eventually you have assimilated the knowledge to the point that you know, almost instinctively, how to apply your knowledge in the action of creating art. This struggle with knowing what action to take, the toil of finding the right technique or method so that what to do next is clear, is at the root of Arjuna's dilemma throughout the entire story of the *Bhagavad Gītā*.

To Arjuna the normal description of meditation made it seem like an arduous and nearly impossible discipline to follow. He said, "The mind is fickle and wavering, as difficult as the wind to control." Also, extended meditation is for people with no responsibilities, no crises, no families to feed, and no cousins and teachers needing to be killed in battle. Kṛṣṇa assures Arjuna that holding the mind in meditation is possible—even in the most difficult situations—through continued practice and non-attachment. Someone who is not connected through to ātman will find yoga difficult, but for one who is united with the ātman, yoga is possible by skillful means. Skillful means, upāya, is the real art of work or practice: it ultimately connects us to the world through the intuitive vision of the ātman. The depth of the whole experience of reality can turn us away from any convoluted preoccupation with our own practice that might sidetrack us. The vision of the ātman can come only when the mind is calm and clear, as in meditation. The techniques of yoga and meditation—the balancing and the counterbalancing, the return to the breath, the gathering together and letting go—are the work. They produce a clear sky in which there is a possibility for insight into the ātman. The insight is not the direct result of any given technique. It is more like an irresistible intuitive sense; the "aha!" of a lighting flash, the unexpected integration and beauty of existence, the vision of the ātman in all beings and of all beings within the ātman. The discipline of meditation is merely an invitation, the accommodating space for the lightning. What ātman is or means must be experienced. It is not just the simple images or concepts of it that we carry in our minds for the convenience of avoiding our circumstances and reassuring our ego.

Even though Arjuna understands this aspect of the ātman, his understanding is not complete, so Kṛṣṇa brings us back into the story by revealing himself personally as the supreme ātman within whom all beings dwell and who is in the heart of all beings. Here the poetic beauty of the *Gītā* unfolds the vision of Kṛṣṇa as everywhere and as all things. In one of the hundreds of verses on how or in what to contemplate the ātman he says, "I am the taste of water; I am the light of the sun and of the moon . . . the sound in the ether . . . the fragrance of the earth," examples that could unfold endlessly. In fact they are doing so now in the world around us. Noticing any of the phenomena pointed out by Kṛṣṇa, having our minds captured by anything that presents itself, and perceiving what we notice in the radically different context of it being the ātman or Kṛṣṇa himself, allows us to see it without the habitual overlay of concepts. Meditation can begin at any of these points. Any of the endless ordinary or extraordinary experiences that we might have can be reframed so that they appear as new and interconnected manifestations of Kṛṣṇa. Phrases like "I am time" or "I am the light in fire" serve as potent mantras to allow us to meditate with close attention on our raw sense experience. The endless manifestations are good news! They give us limitless opportunities to practice the seemingly difficult discipline of meditation.

Having revealed that he (Kṛṣṇa) is all phenomena (even the internal mental qualities that surround Arjuna), he declares that love or bhakti is the heart of the method of yoga and the realization of yoga. These four verses from the tenth chapter are considered to be the core of the *Gītā:*

> I am the source of everything; from Me all flows. Knowing this, the awakened ones [buddhas] endowed with a meditative state, adore Me. Their whole mind enmeshed in Me, their prāṇa going to Me, they are satisfied and they delight in awakening each other and speaking constantly of Me. To them who are constantly linked in yoga, who worship filled with affection, I give the yoga of intelligence [buddhi yoga] by which they come to Me. From compassion for them, I, dwelling in their hearts, destroy the darkness born of ignorance with the shining lamp of knowledge [jñāna]. (X. 8-11)

These verses reveal that it is compassion and surrender that generate the lightning that crosses the gap between us and others, between knowing and the unknowable, between technique and realization.

At this point within the *Gītā*, understanding exactly who and what Kṛṣṇa is becomes even more important. The text goes on with hundreds of examples, saying that he is "all devouring death," that he is, in fact, your very own self, and that his "divine manifestations are infinite." Arjuna, dangling on the edge of realization, is still slightly overwhelmed, if not by his predicament on the battlefield, then at least by the extended personality of his friend and charioteer. The variety of manifestations, explanations, yogas, and things to see are hard to comprehend and remember. At the beginning of the eleventh chapter, Arjuna asks to see Kṛṣṇa's opulent, princely form, his real nature. Perhaps Arjuna was thinking that one form would bind them all and put his own heart at rest.

Kṛṣṇa immediately responds to Arjuna's request—"Just see my hundreds of thousands of divine forms!"—and then he gives to Arjuna an immediate vision of all of the different gods and goddesses that he embodies. He shows Arjuna that he has limitless numbers of mouths and faces, as well as unlimited arms that spread out to infinity. Arjuna is awestruck, noting that all of these are incredibly radiant and bright, as if thousands of suns had arisen simultaneously into the sky. What Arjuna got was a full blow, a direct showing of the expansion of the world process. The teaching was no longer verbal or intellectual but direct and visceral. By letting go of his own story, his own fears and preconceptions, by being blown for an instant into the present moment, Arjuna touches into a true radical mystical experience, which starts to transform his entire existence right from its deepest root. But soon, in the midst of this mystical experience, he becomes confused once again because he begins to analyze, think, and worry. He becomes frightened because he starts to understand that in order to accept the reality of Kṛṣṇa's universal form, he must accept the dissolution of his own immediate, familiar world, his own form; he must let go of his ego. This vision of the universal form, is ultimately the vision of the impermanence, interdependence, and interpenetration of all things. It is the experience of the great matrix of open awareness.

Having become quite distraught and overwhelmed at the sight of Kṛṣṇa's universal forms and with his hair standing up on end from the experience, Arjuna finds himself right back in the same dilemma as at the beginning of the book—sabotaged by his own mind. Again he asks Kṛṣṇa to show him one single but familiar form. Kṛṣṇa obliges and shows Arjuna his form as the god Viṣṇu. Viṣṇu has a beautiful, smiling face, he wears a most elaborate crown and has four arms: one holds a discus, and the others a lotus flower, a mace, and a conch shell. This form of Viṣṇu represents a religion, a social order and a way of life with which Arjuna is familiar, so he begins to relax a little. He thinks that he has "got it," that he can pigeonhole his experience of Kṛṣṇa into the form of Viṣṇu. This of course is comforting to Arjuna, but it again causes him to miss the opportunity to drop deeply into what is actually being presented to him and to truly experience the form. He misses the way these sacred figures of the gods are structured, how their forms are designed to induce a mystical experience. Even though he is more comfortable upon seeing the four-armed form of Viṣṇu in front of him, Arjuna is still not fully relaxed and satisfied. So Kṛṣṇa again reveals his natural form, the medium-sized, normal human form, that is even more familiar—simply Arjuna's old pal Kṛṣṇa. Even though Kṛṣṇa's skin was a stunning dark blue, he is familiar to Arjuna, and Arjuna is finally happy.

This part of the *Bhagavad Gītā* story can be understood in many ways. One interpretation is that what we consider to be ordinary is actually the most sacred of all. There is the story of the student who asked his great teacher, "How big is God," and the teacher replied that god is completely middle sized. It is the nature of mind to interpret our immediate, everyday experience as being too ordinary and too mundane to be sacred. Yet perhaps the most profound, immediate experience of God is an experience of what is happening right here in the present moment. Therefore, that which is arising, which is right in front of our eyes, is to be chosen as the object of meditation, and it is to be observed without comparing it to an idealized form. Sitting in a church and being spontaneously inspired by a ray of light is miraculous, and the same level of deep truth and inspiration could be had while standing in a subway station, reading the newspaper, or arriving at the summit of Mount Kailāsa in the Himalayas. Of course some circumstances are more conducive to inspiring a mystical experience than others, but it is the mind completely merging with *whatever* is arising that allows for that state of mind to arise. At the end of the *Bhagavad Gītā*, Kṛṣṇa explains that the only way for Arjuna to see his final, natural form—Kṛṣṇa's form as Arjuna's best friend, the form with which Arjuna is completely comfortable—is through bhakti, or through love. He points out to Arjuna that this natural form is whatever is appearing right in front of your eyes and elaborates by saying that bhakti is something that is not attainable by following the Vedas or through sacrifice, nor is it attainable by karma yoga, by jñāna yoga, or dhyāna yoga. Bhakti is not hypocritical piety, condescending compassion, or sucrose self-conscious chanting. Bhakti is something beyond methodology; it is merely the nature of pure love.

Another reason that it was difficult for Arjuna, just as it is difficult for us, to see that whatever was in front of his eyes was a form interpenetrated by all other forms, was that such a vision reveals to you—just as Kṛṣṇa revealed to Arjuna—the universal form as the network of your very own body. When we enter the matrix of the body, deep into the central channel, the experience is so vital, so raw and immediate, so joyous, that the mind's ideas about what the world is and its concepts about who we ourselves are fall away because the reality of the universal form is so much more amazing. It is natural for the mind to become terrified by this insight because it (and in particular the part of the mind known as ego) has all kinds of deep hopes and desires that are very well formulated as to its importance in the scheme of who you are. The mind has great plans to torture you for the rest of your life with these ego-centered ideas. If the yogic process actually succeeds in bearing fruit and showing you the nature of reality, then the mind will not be able to make you suffer anymore. Thus as a means of its own survival, the mind is programmed to interpret even a deep mystical experience in such a way as to guarantee that you will never have another one. It is almost as if the mind—for its own survival—*must* play a game of avoidance with profound insight into the nature of reality. Ultimately, calm observation of this game itself becomes a crucial element of a mature yoga practice.

Part of the confusion for Arjuna, as it is for any of us who seek clarity of mind, arises from the fact that there are many approaches, many methods or schools within the system of yoga, that can lead to an enlightened state of being. Within any school of practice there is also always the danger, especially for the narcissist, that the path itself can be turned into a tool for building the ego rather than supporting its dissolution. In fact, within virtually any approach it is far easier for the ego to enhance itself than it is for the methods of the practice to serve their purpose as a means for exposing how the ego functions. This is due to the activity of mind as explained within the Sāṁkhya system: the mind relentlessly creates symbols and images for whatever it is doing, and then the very same mind confuses the symbols it has created for reality or the actual process for which the symbol stands. It is probably the most human and unavoidable temptation to take whatever school of yoga we like and then trivialize or vulgarize it by turning it into an escape—a means of entertainment, a building of the ego, or a means of avoiding reality.

The process by which the mind confuses us into shying away from the mystical experience is that it mistakes the content of our experience with the true nature of the experience itself. This is basic ignorance: we confuse the symbol we associate with the mystical experience for the actual experience. What eventually leads to freedom or to a mystical experience and the taste of enlightenment is not the specifics of the content of your mind but instead the ability to have insight into the vibratory or temporary nature of that content. In this way, any and all content reflects the reality of pure open consciousness and could, therefore, lead to an enlightened state. This insight into the nature of what is arising eventually leads to freedom, to a mystical experience, and to a taste of enlightenment. However, the mind's function is to see and reinterpret the content of thought, so it naturally identifies with specific content then makes a symbol for it, thereby unwittingly short-circuiting the mystical experience in order to do its job well—in order to keep our experiences explainable, categorized, indexed, and useful to the ego.

For example, you go to a church on a bright morning and you sit down in a pew as someone plays Bach on the organ. As you listen, a ray of sunlight streams in through a panel of stained glass. The light reflects on the floor, and suddenly you feel an incredible, endlessly precise sense of harmony. Your hair stands up on end, your tongue is for once quiet, and your inner ear opens to all sounds. You have a mystical experience, the quintessence of the aesthetic experience! Soon thereafter your mind starts to try to understand the experience. It adds up all the information it can about what just happened, and in so doing it identifies the specifics of the experience with the content of the experience. So you walk out of the church and take note, "Oh! That was a Methodist church [or whatever denomination it was]. Then your mind wants to repeat the very same experience by somehow arranging an identical content the next day. The following day you go back to the same church and sit in the same seat next to the same window, and you wait for the same ray of light to pass through the glass and inspire you. What we always discover, however, is that our experience never quite matches our image of the experience, and the precise harmony of the mystical experience we had before eludes us. Even though a perfectly great set of new circumstances might be presenting themselves, conditions that might inspire a completely different form of a mystical experience, we miss the experience because we are waiting for yesterday's circumstances. Waiting for an image of what we imagine the aesthetic experience to be, we miss what is actually arising right under our very own noses that might inspire us anew. We find ourselves again torn by the gap between what is actually arising as our immediate experience and what we think should be arising as our mystical experience. It turns out that as part of a healthy ego function, the mind is programmed to play this very game with the profound insight into the nature of reality. Rather than theorizing about this tendency of mind, instead of trying to squelch it or to get rid of the ego, observing the game itself, without a need to get rid of it, can be the part of the practice that leads to deep insight.

So slippery and cunning are basic ignorance and the ego that they are surrounded and protected by deep irrational emotions. It is the yoga of love, or bhakti, that directly addresses emotions. Deep inside the core of the body lie our very deepest feelings and emotions, and until this depth of our being is addressed, those emotions will act subversively to distract us from genuine practice and from life itself. Left unattended, at some point these deep feelings will sabotage even our most noble endeavors. Bhakti acknowledges all of these profound emotions, and it resolves them through ecstatic love, the nature of which is that you become most happy when the beloved is happy. The real beloved—the actual other being—is outside of the circle of your ego and outside of the categories of your knowledge. When practicing bhakti yoga your own happiness is not the focus of your attention because right at the center of your own being is another being: the beloved. Likewise, at the very, very center of the heart of the beloved is not the beloved, but rather there is another. In the metaphor of the *Bhagavad Gītā*, deep in the very heart of Kṛṣṇa lies everybody else, and Kṛṣṇa becomes ecstatic through making others happy. At the same time, deep in the heart of the devotee is Kṛṣṇa, so the devotee becomes joyous merely by experiencing the delight of Kṛṣṇa. In a sense both are selfless because they have identified with the other at their own core. In bhakti yoga what you find is something like a selfless, perpetual motion machine in which two bright mirrors face each other. As one sees the happiness of the other expanding, one's own happiness blossoms; and when the other apprehends that expansion of happiness in the heart of the other, the other too become ecstatic. The result is an unlimited expansion of consciousness in the form of pure unadulterated joy. This is called ānanda. The word *da* means "to give." So, it is actually by giving to the beloved that happiness comes.

We might question what this pathless path of bhakti or love actually is. The mind, seeing that there is something of great value in bhakti, wants to hold it, to package it, maybe to even sell it. Doing what the mind does best, it reduces the beloved to an image of the beloved. This is exactly what Arjuna wanted: to reduce the universal form of Kṛṣṇa to one single form, when in fact Kṛṣṇa was an unending generation of divine forms. In reducing the beloved to a single form, we become idolaters. In the process of doing so, the most central, liquid current of pure love is extinguished, and we fall back into the mere reflections of what love or bhakti is. Bhakti can very easily degenerate into idolatry and a type of exclusive religious fundamentalism that produces a kind of suppressed disdain and sustained hatred for everybody else except for the beloved—or more accurately, the image of the beloved. Kṛṣṇa is not just a big ego who won the ego game that all beings play. Kṛṣṇa is without "self" at the center of his heart. This lack of self in the supreme Self is ironic, but it is what opens all of the connections of the great network of all beings.

The final teaching that Kṛṣṇa gives to Arjuna is to "abandon in all ways all dharmas and just come to Me as refuge. I will liberate you from all wrongs; do not worry." In other words, let all dharmas be. As we know, dharma has many meanings. In one light it is considered to be religious obligation, duties, and formulations. But dharmas are not just the correct path; they are also the mental factors, the background principles and the elements that create and structure your immediate experience. Give them up, let them go; none of them are absolute. Again, this reflects back and can be understood clearly in light of the Sāṁkhya system's notion that all of the layers of prakṛti are context dependent and empty of a separate self. Earth, water, fire, air, and space are not what are really important. Nor is the buddhi all that important and special. So if you want to *really* do yoga, to give up the patterning of your mind as well as your immediate sense perceptions and feelings, the key is not a technique. The key is merely to accept and trust the essence of love, the essence of your own direct relationship with the beloved. Imagine that Kṛṣṇa was serving Arjuna tea in a cup. The tea is the love, it is the juice, the real message. The cup, of course, is the container. You need the cup in order to serve the scalding hot tea; having it without a cup just does not work. It could be a paper cup or a fancy porcelain cup, whatever serves as the vehicle for delivering the tea will do. Arjuna is fascinated by the container, thinking that the cup is what is important, but Kṛṣṇa tells him, "Taste the tea, Arjuna! Don't worry about the cup." The direct experience of whatever is being presented (in this case the tea) is what is of import. This too is prakṛti, which forms the language, the paper, and the ink for the message. The specific language, the techniques, the forms and images all depend on something else—the context. They will all change, as will the body and the factors that caused prakṛti and the world itself to arise.

"Simply come to me" assumes that one's heart is open and that, therefore, the beloved is very accessible. The teaching of the *Bhagavad Gītā* is not really a formula or a technique, but is instead the teaching that love allows the refinement of a multiplicity of techniques and practices that, like the maṇḍala of prakṛti, fold into each other and transform into the indescribable, ineffable experience of the present moment. It is the teaching of who we really are. The *Bhagavad Gītā* is a fantastic tool—not to be kept on the shelf as an idol but to be read, to be wrestled with, to be reread, consumed, digested, and released.

7

Tantra and the Radiant Earth

> Crying sounds of cuckoos, mating on mango shoots
> Shaken as bees seek honey scents of opening buds,
> Raise fever in the ears of lonely travelers—
> Somehow they survive these days
> By tasting the mood of lovers' union
> In climaxing moments of meditation.
> — *Gītā Govinda* of Jayadeva, I. 36

When we understand that the essence of yoga is that of pure love, pure bhakti, it is natural to think that this is exactly what we want to do; to give up everything else and discover pure love. But then we find ourselves wondering how to actually go about doing so using our body and mind. Even though the senses and the mind may have given us a flash of insight into the teaching of bhakti, we are confounded by the task of deciding exactly what action to take in order to act in a way that reflects pure love. So the mind does what it does best: it begins to categorize, theorize, attach itself to ideas, and as it does this we encounter the danger of feeding our own ego as we imagine we are following the path of yoga. Using the mind, the senses, and the ego to realize yoga is like asking a bull to fix the porcelain it just knocked off the shelf; there is a very real danger that the bull will make an even greater mess. In our practice of yoga, however, we have no choice but to use ourselves as we search for insight.

The true practice of yoga cannot occur until all aspects of experience throughout the day and night are attended to with singular intention and devotion. All of the things that you do, everything that constitutes real life can be yoga. Otherwise our actions and the events of our life become distractions and pockets in which the ego can hide. For example, cooking and eating can become part of the practice or a great escape from it. Imbalanced eating, from gorging with junk food to punishing the body with a salad diet, is a common and effective way for the ego to sabotage yoga. Alternatively, food can be selected, handled, and prepared as if it were a way of benefiting or communicating with the beloved, a means of connecting sensually with pure awareness directly through your taste buds. The practice becomes one in which while tasting food you might think, "The beloved within me is tasting this offering through me, and the food itself is the supreme deity." The same concentration and awareness can be brought to walking, running, working, thinking, and even to pleasures like love and relaxation. This same depth of devotion can be carried out with every breath, every thought, and in every situation when practicing yoga. When we find that our need to practice yoga and meditation has come to every aspect of the inner and outer worlds, the time is here to dip into the vast ocean of what is called tantra—the experiential unveiling of reality.

Tantra is one of those exciting buzzwords that catches the ear and invokes images of the sensual, exotic, and the mysterious. Complex occult rituals, magic spells, and touching the dark side of things are associated with tantra. Yet a broad look at the many schools, practices, and philosophies of tantra show a bright and beautiful side, essential for a yoga student to know. Tantra means extending a thread or a weaving of threads; it also implies the stretching out on a loom of connections in order to form an interpenetrating network or a matrix. Tantra forms a vast complex of specific practices and rituals done in endless detail to sanctify every particular of our experience. Within the matrix of tantric practices the worship of feminine deities is dominant, since in Vedic culture the main deities were male deities. Tantra not only rhymes with, but its meaning overlaps with that of the words *mantra* and *yantra*. Mantras are vibrant chants that bring us into heightened awareness and concentration; yantras are geometric forms, which are drawn or visualized to aid concentration. Within the various schools of tantra we do not find any unique philosophical point of view, nor do we find any idea that is not already expounded upon in other more orthodox schools. Hence it is difficult to explain the history of tantra. In a sense it can be said that tantra is a composite of all of those practices and views that are on the borderline between various yoga philosophies. It has become the language of exchange between different schools of practice.

like an inspired tapestry tantra weaves a web Quivering & life + desire

Thousands of years ago in the age of the early Upaniṣads and of the Buddha, there were many people practicing yoga, experimenting with different techniques and various approaches in order to understand the meaning of reality. Gradually these methods evolved into schools of philosophical understanding as practitioners discussed their practices, their philosophies, and experiences—perhaps in the marketplace or over a meal. It was in that world, where the schools actually met each other—in the alleys between the various ashrams—that tantra flowed. Tantra is like a lingua franca, the currency of exchange between schools. It is where practice and experience count, where the concern is not so much to establish a historical school, a cult, or a religion that dominates others. Instead tantra is the basket from which various schools of philosophy and practice arise, just as it is the ocean into which all of this variety of practice and thought eventually returns. There is a natural evolution that occurs within the process of all philosophical thinking: as the streams of thought deepen and the ideas ripen, different schools appear to accommodate the innovative insights at hand. Sometimes, because the ideas are so complex and rich, even perhaps controversial, new systems evolve into secret, occult, diverse schools of practice in the same way tantric practices and thought have evolved within the yoga tradition. As is true with most of these offshoot schools, including tantra, to an outsider some of the practices and streams of thought may seem extreme or outlandish. However, tantric ideas are not designed for their eccentricity; rather they are constructed to be fully absorbing as a means of bringing every ounce of practitioners' attention into *+ experience*

using

the essence, the juice, of whatever is arising before them. If you meet someone who is a truly devout tantric, you will discover a practitioner uniquely themselves, fully enmeshed in the world, fully focused with a dedication to just doing the practices as a method of tapping into the deep beauty and joy of liberation for themselves and for others. This form of awakening is the nectar, the juice, of real tantric practice.

Within Indian philosophy the term *rasa* is used when describing nectar of the aesthetic experience. *Rasa,* which literally means "juice" or "essence," refers to relationships between people and things and to the different moods and types of beauty and joy that are formed. The different rasas serve to absorb the mind into deep meditation. A very tangible and literal experience of rasa flows out of the different sacrifices and pūjās performed for the pleasure of the deities in temples. In these rituals the priests chant, offer incense, and bathe statues of the deities in mixtures of milk, honey, water, yogurt, and other liquids. Having flowed over the deity, the liquids are then a sacred drink. This rasa, which sometimes is channeled to flow in a spout out of the temple, is collected so that the devotees may drink it as part of their practice. Tantra is often considered equivalent to this ritualistic rasa, because in its higher forms it focuses on the direct aesthetic experience and the

Nectar from the Moon (6)

One of the meanings of the word *rasa* is "relationship," referring to the aesthetic pleasure coming from interfacing with another. The different rasas, or flavors, of love correspond to a strong feeling of luminous, intense, pleasurable joy, which seems to come from what is called the root of the palate. The root of the palate is located approximately at the pituitary gland, and is felt by releasing the soft palate as if subtly smiling. The quintessence of all of the rasas is called *amṛta*, or nectar. Its primary quality is compassion. The nectar drips down through the petals of the sahasrāra, the thousand-petaled lotus, to the reservoir just above the root of the palate called the moon. When mūla bandha, or yoni mudrā, is done well it causes nectar to drip from this moon and that nectar fills all of the nāḍīs, transforming one's body and every sensation into the experience of consciousness and joy.

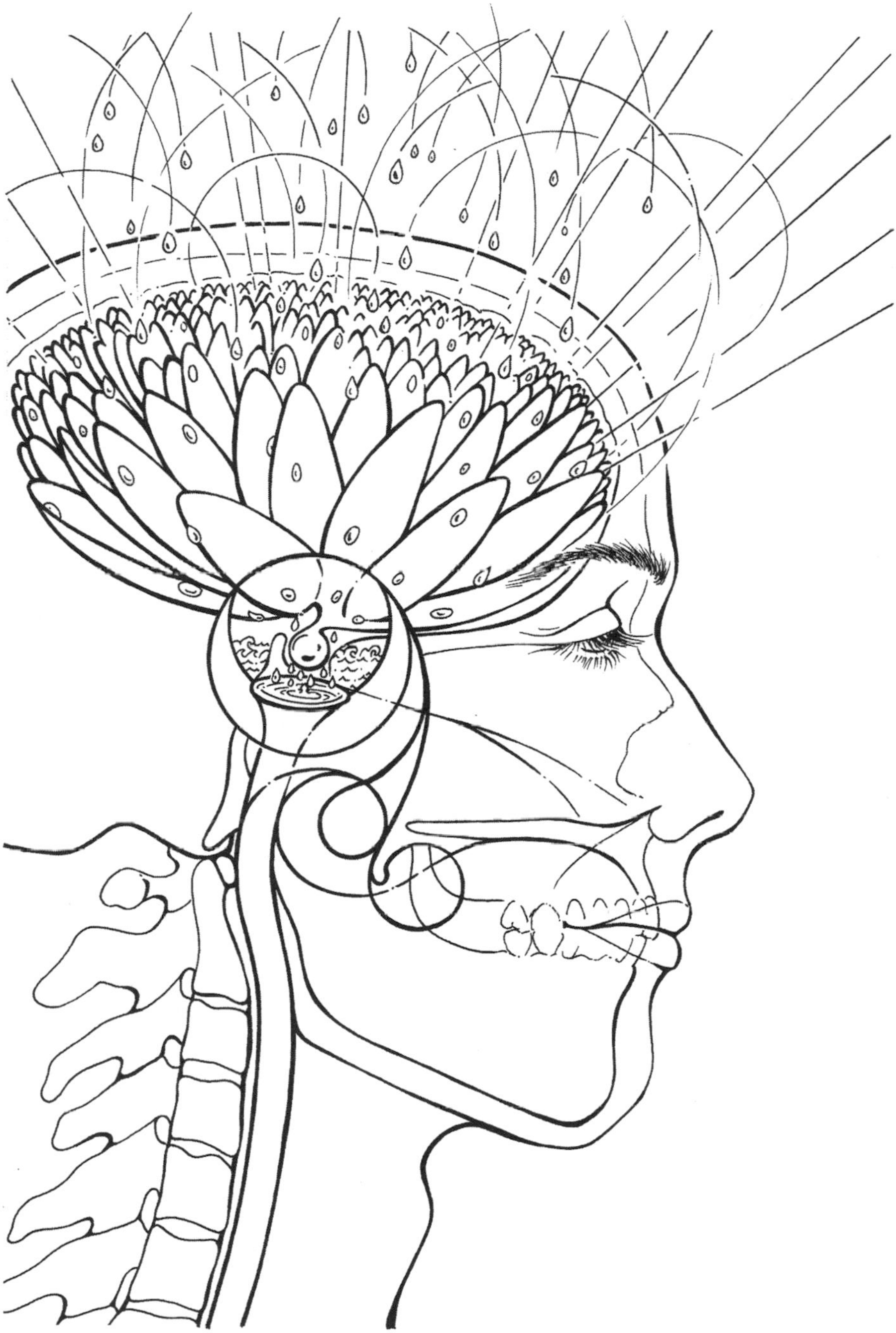

metaphorical juice of ecstatic concentrated emotions generated from successful practices and meditations. The nature of all liquid, of course, is that it will take on the shape of whatever container in which it is held, but the liquid itself is not actually the shape of the container. So tantric philosophies and practices are simply containers for the delivery of the rasa, in essence the love, which is the nectar of liberation that flows forth through an authentic practice. This elixir—enlightenment—is actually what tantra is concerned with.

Taking a somewhat broader view we find that the teachings of haṭha yoga are actually tantric. In fact, it is said in the *Haṭha Yoga Pradīpikā* that the kuṇḍalinī, the awakening of the power of the internal breath into the central channel of the body, is the foundation of all tantra. Since the underlying focus of tantra is this visceral experience of the present moment, tantric practices always remain something of a secret because the truth that lives in the central channel is subtle, elusive, and ultimately something each of us can experience only for ourselves. If we concur that the secret of tantra is to pay attention to what is actually arising in the present moment, then the mind says, "Oh! That sounds very simple" until we attempt to pay attention to what is actually occurring. Immediately we find that the conceptualizing mind, which is always externalizing experience by making theories, is unable to actually watch what is arising. The deep process that tantra taps into is an absorption of mind to the point that it can simply observe, without interfering, that which is unfolding. Tantra works, therefore, by ritualizing ordinary day-to-day sensual and mental experiences (sometimes in excruciatingly precise detail and degree) in order to stimulate and focus the mind, free of theory, on the immediate arising of feelings, thoughts, and sensations within any experience. By learning to tap small currents of rasa, derived from the skillful joining of opposites, there is a releasing of things and objects of the senses into their background. The practice is ultimately the same as in yoga and Sāṁkhya, but a tantric metaphor for practice would revolve around pleasurable juice extraction as opposed to merely mindful observation.

For example, through the use of mudrā, or the joining together of the fingers or hands into precise patterns (which is a classic tantric ritual), you can visualize and experience fully the divine goddess. You can imagine your thumbs as being different aspects of the body of the deity and through mantras and meditations on the sensations of your two thumbs touching, a connection to whatever is arising within your consciousness spontaneously occurs. The meditation can then be deepened through concentrating on the tips of the forefingers, middle, ring, and little fingers. The focus might then spread to the centers of the palms and deep into the nervous system, as through the practice you begin to ritualize various points of contact and the sensations throughout the entire body. All of these are simply techniques to help you wake up to the foremost secret that is right in front of your eyes all the time: that the world as it is being presented to us right here, right now is utterly sacred and mysterious. Our body and the world are the divine body and mind of the goddess. Through tantra and other forms of yoga we learn that paying close attention to whatever is arising reveals its inscrutable depths and leaves us in a state of awe with insight into the nature of mind and reality.

A popular metaphor in tantra is that of the play and interpenetration of the god Śiva and his consort Śakti. Their coming together is the basis of all experience and indeed of the whole of creation. Unlike the formal dualism in Sāṁkhya, a variety of different schools of nondualism allow Śiva and Śakti, Kṛṣṇa and Rādhā, and even puruṣa and prakṛti, to be two aspects of one pure consciousness. Then from being pure, free, contentless consciousness, Śiva penetrates and shines through Śakti. They appear as layered between each other, reacting to and inspiring one another. Each is selfless and is always finding his or her self in the other. They form mirrors of each other, and their relationship is the purest bhakti. They can be felt tangibly in our bodies as the interplay of prāṇa and apāna, the spin and counterspin that prāṇa and apāna produce in our limbs and our āsana practice. Prāṇāyama and āsana are both perfected when we let prāṇa and apāna squeeze together and interpenetrate in this kind of affectionate union.

One of the axiomatic truths of all yogic and tantric practices is that we must use the same ground upon which we have fallen in order to stand up, and as we know, the mind, which is so deeply the cause of our suffering, must use itself to relieve our own misery. Tantric practices are one means of seeing through this suffering by facing the avidyā, or the ignorance, that wrongly perceives reality through dualistic mental filters. These practices help us to recognize our tendency to confuse that which is permanent with the temporary forms that manifest within our mind. Of course we must use the mind in order to wake up out of the field of avidyā, and so tantric practices are designed to spread out the whole spectrum of the imagination and the emotions, and then to engage the mind in any and all of its aspects with a sharp, penetrating focus, so that the present circumstances can be experienced directly as the interpenetration of Śiva and Śakti. This automatically brings relief from the suffering because it allows the mind to follow a thread of insight deep into the core of reality.

Tantric practices are deliberately constructed to use form and language in this way, as a means of focusing the mind so that it can use itself—its own perceptions—to stand up and awaken from the ignorance of confusion. Constructions of mind can be seen with utter clarity because even the simplest function of life or the tiniest detail are considered to be the very center of experience. Experience is observed, faced, and penetrated with intelligence; there is no turning from or denying of it. Through the practices we are able to experience the forms of the mind as empty, as having no permanent structure; we experience all form as sacred and specific forms as pure radiance. This is why one of the characteristics of tantric schools is that they become involved in such tiny details, so that everything can be momentarily pulled out of and then threaded back into the full matrix of its background. Each particular, unique thing interpenetrates and shines through all other unique and particular things. This too is the ideal vision of the divine body of the goddess. Tantric rituals are excellent methods for drawing us into the present moment, but because of their focus on detail the tantric schools also have the potential to become lost in the concept and particulars of form.

When you mention the word *tantra* in India, many people will raise their eyebrows and give you a disapproving look at the mere thought that you even know the word. This is because the vast study of tantra has not only the deepest insights that fulfill the purposes of the Vedas, the Upaniṣads, and the *Yoga Sūtra*, but also some practices that can easily be (and often are) misused and abused. For example, over the course of time some tantric practices have evolved to include recitation of mantra and the contemplation of yantra for the accumulation of power and personal sensual experience, without any concern for others or for the practices' true significance within the bigger scheme of reality. In the modern world we have to recognize the vague, secretly erotic, illicit, exploitive, ungrounded sense that is invoked when we use the word *tantra*. Due to its misuse, today the idea of tantra can conjure up images of sexual orgies or of exotic, repulsive practices and rituals. Many tantric practices are done from an egocentric perspective, out of context and without a teacher. The yogic context of the practices is to examine closely every corner of life—even normally taboo and repressed corners—so as to embrace rather than deny the shadow sides of our own mental constructions.

It is a shame that tantra is sometimes reduced to its eye-catching aspects, because higher and deeper tantra looks on everything within our experience as sacred and as part of an interrelated matrix of experience and understanding. The misperceptions of tantra arise in part because it specifically looks on those things we typically do not like to look at (or things our culture does not like to look at) as being sacred. Consequently, tantric practices often involve the extreme realms of the mind and the senses. We find within Indian mythology various deities, goddesses and gods, involved in exciting stories of extreme violence or extreme passion. For instance, there is the image of a goddess with skulls dangling around her neck, which could easily be perceived as demonic or wildly exotic. In fact the skulls are often considered symbolic of the letters of the alphabet, indicating that the goddess has severed words from their objects and meanings, thereby liberating us (and the objects) from the maze of language that reduces objects to mind-constructed names and thoughts about them. Ultimately you could say that tantra examines those parts of our mind and our existence that we do not want to face: the foremost of these being impermanence and selflessness. For example, there are stories of the vast slaughter of beings, which in fact is

skulls around kali's neck = letters of alphabet

something that the universe is actually engaged in and also something most of us do not like to dwell on. But if we step back and take a look at the process of time, we see that the universe, from certain points of view, is a giant death machine, an unending slaughter of beings from which no one will escape. All the emotions and all the aversions and fears that the mind can generate when we contemplate this idea of death—or any other aspect of life that is difficult to face—are drawn out within Indian mythology and within tantric practice so that we can experience the entire potential of our own imagination without superimposing theory onto it.

This process of bringing attention to even the most unpleasant aspects of what is arising is also something we do in our everyday yoga practice as we work with āsana within the realm of feeling and sensation. We explore and open the joints of the body, we uncover fields of sensation and tone, and we expose our deepest emotions in order to experience them without attachment. In this way we open up all the realms of experience and the fields of potential in the mind, just as we would fan out a deck of cards. The effect is that the mind is stunned as it momentarily drops its presuppositions; we become free of the imagination and liberated from the heavy hand of dominance of the ego within the mind. In that instant, when the yoga is working, we can actually have a direct experience of reality. Tantric yoga practices in particular allow us to explore the extremes of the imagination, from the most positive and heavenly to the most negative and hellish. So even though some might prefer to think of tantra as exclusively a means of exploring the world of sexuality, this of course is just one corner of what it is about. Since sexuality is sublimated in so many cultures, and because sexual practices can free the mind from its thinking function, the tantric notion of experiencing reality through the present moment could translate into the misperception that tantra means only sex. Tantric rituals were considered by some ancient scholars as the best method for sublimating and also for fulfilling the immense power and urge that embodied beings have toward sexual fulfillment, and indeed sexual awareness is integral to any disciplined practice of yoga that addresses the body fully. In fact, as we go deeply into hatha yoga through āsana, prāṇāyāma, and meditation, we are tapping into our own sexual energy as we touch the prāṇa in the core of the body. If this energy is denied, it can come back and sabotage even a sincere yogi in subtle or gross ways. This same prāṇa, or pattern of sensation, branches through many levels of desire, attachment, and imagination as it constructs our world experience so that if it is unresolved at a deep sexual level, the very same prāṇa can move the mind in devious ways.

The misperception that tantra is exclusively a group of practices having to do with sexuality also stems from the fact that yoga involves the awakening of the power of the serpent kuṇḍalinī, which is imagined coiled up and asleep, blocking the opening of the central channel. When awakened she uncoils, opening the mouth of the central channel; she then turns around and enters the suṣumnā. Her movement in this central channel, the middle path of the subtle body, causes the mind, the citta, to drop into deepening layers of profound meditation. There is an obvious parallel between the sexual potential that rests within the body and the presence and awakening of this serpent that dwells above the center of the pelvic floor. This coiling of the sexual energy, which is the normal state for most people, blocks the central channel and causes us to project our sexual desires externally onto sense objects. The citta (mind and intelligence), which follows the prāṇa, also then coils and superimposes symbols onto processes, creating in the mind the appearance of separate sense objects. In this light we can see that kuṇḍalinī represents more than just sexual desire; she is also the desire to know things, the craving not to suffer, and the aspiration for liberation for oneself and for all others. A balanced study and practice of yoga brings attention to the true nature of others and the mind, and to how many aspects of life are interconnected. An unbalanced, exclusive focus on obscure tantric practices having to do with uncoiling our sexual energy, without proper grounding in the truth of impermanence, may put us in the situation of being obsessed by imaginary powers and ruled by the ego. There are high intoxicated states of mind in which we still split desire, sensation, and feeling into subject and object. The subject-object divide revolves around the ego and stems from the primordial ignorance (avidyā), which has gotten us into this situation in the first place.

Kundalini represents the desire to know things

In the skilled practice of tantric yoga there is the awakening of internal energy and an experience of the full intensity of sensation and feeling we term *sexuality*. In that awakening, when the practice is balanced, there is a release of the ego's tendency to grasp onto the division of subject and object, so that the cause of great frustration and suffering does not occur.

One of the teachings of the Bhagavad Gītā is that kāma, which means "lust," is considered to be a great sin and an immense enemy because it inevitably causes hatred or anger. Intense emotions typically arise from a state of lust because it is an ego-based mind state that represents an absolute split between subject and object. Due to this division, it is virtually impossible to fulfill the kind of endless desire that arises from lust, and the residue from that lack of fulfillment results in cycles of confusion and delusion. In fact, it is the nature of ego that it can never be truly satisfied or fulfilled, no matter how much enjoyment and gratification it gets. A deep sense of satisfaction is accessible only when the union of opposites is perceived, when the interpenetration of foreground with background is experienced. As such, since by definition the ego is separate from all else, it can never be completely fulfilled. The practices of yoga and of tantra cultivate the complete reversal of the tendencies of mind and ego to split things into subjects and objects. Proper practice does not try to eliminate desire; it eliminates the perception of their being a subject and object. So practice opens a source of unending and lasting contentment and pleasure through the realization of desire without projecting that desire onto any object. Kuṇḍalinī, the summation of deep desire on many levels, awakens from her coil in the pelvic floor and flows on the middle path to her true love Śiva, or pure consciousness, at the crown of the head. The goddess kuṇḍalinī is of course prakṛti from the Sāṁkhya system, and Śiva is puruṣa. Yoga is then total satisfaction and complete pleasure within the present moment without the ego; without the self (the ultimate subject) trying to define and then grasp or reject an object that it perceives as separate.

In tantric yoga it is postulated that the awakening of the kuṇḍalinī stimulates an immensely satisfying flow of joy and pleasure and of deep emotion far more profound than any feeling or sentiment we can think about or describe. The awakening allows a quality of awareness that is neither conceptual nor imagined to flourish so that perceptions become immediate, essential, vibrant, and living. Without the arousing of this energy deep in the core of the body, there is more potential for fantasy, an element of unmet desire or of intellectualization arising at the core of your yoga practice. This is because the body holds the history of our mental activities within its habitual patterns, in muscles and connective tissues as well as in habits of perception and movement. The closing verse of the *Haṭha Yoga Pradīpikā* summarizes this: "As long as the prāṇa has not entered to flow in the middle path and the bindu droplet does not become firm from binding the prānic winds; as long as the mind does not assume the form of effortless spontaneous arising, all talk of wisdom is unfounded prattle and nonsensical hypocrisy."

Another important aspect of tantra is that it deliberately uses what you might call a "gross-out factor" as a method of bringing awareness into clear focus. In other words, tantric teachings often include practices that focus on facets of ordinary life that are not usually dealt with, sometimes not even acknowledged in proper society. For instance, for many people it is virtually impossible to grasp and deal with the fact that we will all die and that the body we so dearly love and identify with will become disfigured, decompose, and transform into what might be considered a disgusting state. This unavoidable dissolution of the body can cause great fear and avoidance. In order to face this part of reality and to not separate subject and object in a pattern of fear, rejection, and avoidance when considering death, some schools of tantra actually encourage students to locate dead bodies—dig them up if they are buried or find them before they are cremated—and to sit on the corpse for meditation. There are mantras and offerings that are specifically prescribed for the charnel grounds. The Vedic fire sacrifice is given a nice twist as the body itself is considered to be the best and most complete offering into the sacred cremation fire. Some tantrics will actually even engage in eating the flesh of the dead body. These practices are carried out not for the sole purpose of revolting the practitioner or anyone unlucky enough to be watching, but as a means of demonstrating and contemplating impermanence and mentally constructed perceptions of the nature of most of our preferences and repulsions. This is only one small example of how some tantric practices initially appear quite extreme. They are powerful as a means of focusing the mind, ridding it of its preconceptions, and as a method of facilitating the dissolving of ego.

A well-known practice within tantric yoga is called the pañcamakāra, or the five *m*'s. The five *m*'s are: madya, which means "wine" or "alcoholic beverage"; māṁsā, which means "meat"; matsya, meaning "fish"; mudrā, which means "parched grains," "toasted grains as an aphrodisiac," "a seal which presses opposites together" (or within Buddhist tantra it means a sexual partner); and finally maithuna, meaning "sexual intercourse." For members of proper Hindu society, engaging in some of these five activities is considered taboo and even thinking about them creates a certain queasy feeling. Within what is called the left-handed schools of tantric practice, wine is ingested and meat and fish are ritualistically eaten—which can be intense if you are vegetarian as many Hindus are. The idea of mudrā or pressing is practiced either as eating grain or by experiencing the presence of a sexual partner. This is followed at the end of the rite by engaging in sexual intercourse. Usually the pañcamakāra practice is not looked upon lightly; the activities are carried out ritualistically with great care and the use of many, many mantras. Though it can be a very formal practice, it can be done with lighthearted ease. Even within most left-handed schools of tantra there is usually very little sense of debauchery. The ritual is carefully designed to prevent our habit of reducing other people and ourselves to our theories about them.

For people in modern society who eat meat or fish on a regular basis, who drink wine with every meal, and who have been exposed to sexual practices since their early teens, there is very little gross-out factor with the pañcamakāra practice. Indulging in the five *m*'s for some is like a standard Friday night out, so the tantric effect is not quite the same for them as it would be for a devout Hindu. Perhaps for modern people a different type of five *m*'s ritual could be established. This of course would involve finding things that for us have an equally engaging sensual quality to them but that are somewhat taboo; tantric sexual rituals for someone who engages in sexual activity regularly would have to have a twist to them. Many of us who equate tantra with sex might assume that simply having excessive amounts of sex, attending orgies, or performing sex in unusual manners is the equivalent of participating in a tantric practice. However, a truly tantric practice might mean having sex with a sexual partner whom you are not particularly attracted to, or if you consider yourself a highly sexual person, it might even mean abstaining from sex altogether. Within tantric yoga there is the reversing of taboos, making you cross lines that are not only boundaries that society has laid down, but also lines that your own mind has drawn. Stepping over this type of line has a very potent effect and can practically drive you crazy if you are not fully conscious and if you do not keep your ego at bay. At the same time, these types of practices can induce or offer the opportunity to have a profoundly deep core experience about the nature of your own mind and your own reality if you remain centered and clear.

Many schools of tantra are considered to be right-handed, meaning that the practitioners are celibate or married and are usually very conservative people within those contexts. A right-handed tantric would consider the five *m*'s practice as something that can be practiced symbolically as a means of waking up the internal process of yoga. Accomplished yoga practitioners consider deep internal experiences to be that which is most exciting, and practicing a symbolic version of the five *m*'s would suffice to open the senses and the mind. It is interesting to note that celibate monks feel compassion for those who must practice the external five *m*'s in order to get any sense of the nature of the internal experience. It is also true that many tantrics feel sorry for celibate monks.

One extraordinarily beneficial effect of tantric practices is that they are designed to make you relax and let go; they teach the skill of leaving things alone just as they are. Tantra can reveal that reality is at the same time more subtle and complex than the mind can ever know, and that it is also far more beautiful and deep than can be imagined. The practices disclose the mind as simply one aspect of truth, and they demonstrate that the mind can neither embrace nor control life. So for the average yoga practitioner tantra is good news; it is essentially a method for presenting the perspective that life is wonderful, ecstatic, and that by its very nature it is pure joy. Tantra also allows us to look at the deeply horrible aspects of existence. It addresses the face of impermanence, the fact of death, degeneration, and ultimately the end of the cosmos. Through tantra we can look at all of this—both the joyous and the terrifying aspects of life—without grasping at them or shrinking away from them, and also without any sense of unmet desire or fear. Tantric practices reveal those things that may be considered the most horrible aspects of life, or the most blissful and intimate, those things that should never even be talked about publicly (especially with children) as a cause of great happiness. Tantra allows us to perceive and to merge with the full spectrum of life as it really is. It allows us to arrive fully within each yoga practice so that we are free of the extremes of idealism and perfectionism. Perhaps the most wonderful gift of tantra is that it underscores the sense that, in all aspects of life, we are entering a matrix that is like the arms of a great loving mother where we can be totally happy and completely at peace without having to *be* something or *know* something. Tantra becomes a method for insight into the core teachings of yoga and into the realization that things are quite interesting just as they are right here in the present moment.

8

THE *YOGA SŪTRA*

NOT MUCH IS KNOWN about the actual history of the sage Patañjali, the composer of the *Yoga Sūtra*. Tradition considers him to be an incarnation of the divine serpent Ādi Śeṣa, the primordial residue, who has an unlimited number of heads and one tail. This same serpent serves as the couch of the god Visnu and all creation—the world—and incarnates in supporting roles whenever needed. Ādi Śeṣa is the archetype of the well-aligned yoga posture as well as the residue used as the material of meditation in deep samādhi. The name *Patañjali* means "fallen from prayer" or "fallen from praying hands." One story would have it that when his mother picked up her newborn son in her hands, she was so shocked by his serpentine half that she accidentally dropped him; he fell from her praying hands. In any case the Yog*a Sūtra* has been so useful and penetrating in its explanations of the yoga path that people consider the author to be truly divine.

It is believed by many scholars that the *Yoga Sūtra* was composed at around 250 B.C.E. This was after the arising of the Mahāyāna school of Buddhism, in which there was a strong emphasis on compassion and on the nondual doctrine of emptiness. We find within the text of the *Yoga Sūtra* many, many terms that are uncommon within the yoga tradition yet which work well when cross-referenced with Buddhism. This in and of itself is very interesting because it is a demonstration of how the thinkers within the yogic and Buddhist systems were in contact with and were influencing one another. The *Yoga Sūtra* begins with the phrase "atha yoga anuśāsanam," which translates as "now the exposition of yoga." The word *atha* means "now," and in this case it refers to the present moment, to the here and now. Beginning the *Yoga Sūtra* with the word *now* implies that we have finally come to a point where we are ready to inquire into the truth and achieve a direct experience of it. It also implies that we have already tried everything else we can think of as a means of relieving suffering—we have tried sex, drugs, and rock and roll, religion, piety, and self-improvement seminars. None of it has truly worked, so now we are finally ready to investigate the root cause of suffering and to explore the methods and the path for eliminating that suffering.

The next aphorism that Patañjali gives is a brief and useful definition of yoga: "Yoga is the cessation of the turnings of the mind" (yogaḥ citta vṛtti nirodhaḥ). The term *nirodha* is interpreted in many different ways. In fact it is good while studying the *Yoga Sūtra* to explore the various possibilities of meaning for the different sūtras presented in the numerous commentaries written by various scholars over the centuries. Nirodha can mean to make still the presentations in the mind, or it can mean the release of the agitation of mind. It can also mean the complete cessation of the presentations of the mind, implying that some of the states of deep yoga are experiences beyond thought and beyond thought construction. When this stillness of mind occurs, it is said that then the seer (which is actually pure consciousness, or in Sāṁkhya terminology, the puruṣa) stands free in its own form. In other words, there is no identification of the seer with that which is seen, that is, the constructions of the mind (the prakṛti). This is said to be the initial state or flash of enlightenment or liberation. In all other states—when the mind is looping with vṛttis—there is misperception and an identification by the seer with whatever is arising in the mind. When this happens the natural tendency is for the mind to drop into a state of grasping for or pushing away whatever it is identifying with, depending on the perceived value of the presentation in relation to the ego.

These looplike turnings of the citta, when not suspended or seen through in yoga, prevent the natural, radiant nature of pure awareness from unfolding; their misperception is the root cause of great suffering. Patañjali describes two categories for these loopings of the citta. Those that cause torment and suffering are called kliṣṭa. Others are called akliṣṭa; they are neutral and do not cause torment and suffering. This is an extremely important point made right at the beginning of the *Yoga Sūtra*. Many citta vṛttis are important and needed as props for meditation and as the content of intelligent thought. The tormenting vṛttis often cease thanks to the background work of those that are nontormenting. By the same token, the nontormenting vṛttis are absolutely necessary as well, and they too drop their structures and forms in deeper states of meditation. Yoga actually improves the thinking process rather than creating a catatonic state. It is important to remember that even though the deeper practices of yoga lead to states of mind in which thought comes to a point of cessation, yoga is not an antithought practice. Instead it is the refinement of the art of thinking, allowing chains of thought to unfold within an open sky of compassion and intelligence. Rather than just giving up with an attitude of, "well, thought has gotten us into all of this trouble so now we are not going to think at all," yoga encourages clear, penetrating thinking. It is astonishing how frequently and easily this has been misinterpreted over the centuries by those unwilling to enjoy the paradoxes of thought that are revealed and observed within a healthy yoga practice.

In the next sūtra of the first pāda (chapter) the five types of vṛttis or mind processes are defined. The first is pramāṇa, true perception. These are thoughts that are correct and clear thinking, that form truthful, honest propositions about the world. Pramāṇa is associated with accurate direct perception, unambiguous logical thinking, and accepting testimony from reliable others. In contrast, viparyaya, wrong perception, is seen as misconception, misperception, or simply mistaken thought and theory. Viparyaya is a proposition formulated on misunderstanding of either external or internal phenomena. It is crucial to understand the distinction between pramāṇa and viparyaya. Both types of thought are citta vṛttis, yet as their definition indicates, not all thoughts are equally sound, nor are all thoughts equally accurate and precise. It is very important to be able to see things clearly within the practice of yoga, and if one does come up with a wrong concept, it is vitally important to be able to discover the confusion and to correct the misperception through intelligent investigation.

The next vṛtti described in the *Yoga Sūtra* is the mind state called vikalpa. *Kal* means "to imagine," *vi* means "to divide"; *vikalpa*, then, means "divided imagination." This is simply the way the mind constructs its experience through what can be described as imagination or a combining of images and perceptions in the thought process, without any correspondence to any established substance or phenomena. Sometimes vikalpa is also used to describe the entire process of the world and the mind. From this point of view, vikalpa is all divided construction and as such is part of all mental creations, even the correct perceptions. Comprehending the idea of vikalpa is essential if we are to understand the description, within the *Yoga Sūtra*, of how the mind works with imagination at the root of all other states of mind, all the other vṛttis. The imagination is so vast and so deep that the mind easily becomes embroiled by it, especially if there is not a clear understanding of the mind's tendency toward vikalpa, or divided construction.

Sleep, or nidrā, is considered to be the fourth type of vṛtti. Deep sleep and the dream state can be completely absorbing, so they are sometimes confused with the state of samādhi (absorption) or with the state of nirodha (cessation of the agitation of mind). In samādhi the mind is alert and awake; sleep, however, usually blocks these more radiant states. Unlike samādhi, a state of deep sleep is characterized by a very strong inertia, which is accompanied by strong physical sensations that keep pulling on and dissolving the mind rather than making it vital and alert. When one is beginning a yoga practice, nidrā can also be confused with a state of samādhi. You fall asleep while sitting in meditation, and you think, "Wow, that was certainly peaceful, I must have experienced samādhi!" But this type of dullness is not actually what yoga is all about. Yoga is an extraordinarily brilliant, calm, and intelligent state of awakeness. In fact, the very meaning of the word *buddhi* (intelligence) is to continually awaken from different shelves of awareness. Yoga is always a process of awakening and then waking up again out of the storylike loopings of the mind into the present moment.

The final vṛtti described in the *Yoga Sūtra* is smṛtayaḥ, or memory. Smṛtayaḥ indicates deep memories, memories that could go back within our own life, even to our childhood, or perhaps, within the scheme of the transmigration of the subtle body, smṛtayaḥ could be considered a memory that reaches from one life to another. Within this type of deep memory there is the opportunity to understand the entire patterning of one's conditioning, and through the practice of meditation to become deconditioned from the restraints that patchy, unexamined memory imposes. Memory relates to deep core feelings as conditioning in the prāṇa; it holds many of our unconscious attitudes, anxieties, and fears. Becoming mindful of smṛtayaḥ allows the opportunity to actually make associations with our present experience, and the awareness facilitates insight into how we are programmed by associations that link back to past experience. Smṛtayaḥ allows us to let go of chains of past experience and thought that have led to faulty perception and misinterpretation of reality in the present moment. This clarification of the layers within memory is accomplished through meditation practice and by observing whatever is arising just as it is without meddling—without attempting to change or fix anything, without grasping or pushing away the memory.

The five types of vṛttis are said to be either miserable or painful (kliṣṭa), or they are considered to be not miserable or not painful in nature (akliṣṭa). When you are engaged in the practice of yoga, the vṛttis themselves (whether miserable or not) become stepping-stones for the practice. They become objects upon which to meditate without attachment, and as such they are extremely useful. When the presentation in the mind, the vṛtti, is made stable by simply observing it through a meditative quality of mind, then you are able to examine the vṛtti clearly, and in that examination you may be able to experience its true nature as something that is sacred. When it links into its background, into its immediate contexts, when it stretches on and on, connecting into everything, we can say that it is sacred. With this shift in perspective there is a natural release of the vṛtti, and in that release the insight of yoga begins. Eventually we are able to see that all states of mind, all states of being, everything that arises, is sacred. This insight into the nature of reality naturally brings us to a state of nirodha; we come into a state in which the agitation of the mind automatically ceases, as if we were stunned and awestruck by the depth, beauty, and simplicity of the ātman.

We learn from the *Yoga Sūtra* that nirodha is reached through the twofold process of abhyāsa and vairāgyam. Abhyāsa means the effort to practice in the sense of sticking with a repeating or replicating pattern. Through the repetition of a pattern that frames and reframes the content of the mind, a close observation of the content that can lead to nirodha is possible. Abhyāsa includes all the efforts of collecting together mind and body through yoga āsana, meditation, chanting, and prāṇāyāma, so that the workings of the mind are revealed. The other end of the stick that leads to nirodha is the practice of vairāgyam, or of letting go, of nonattachment. Once we see the patterns within the mind, rather than trying to change, fix, or alter them in any way, we simply allow the patterns to be; that is vairāgyam. We do not ignore the patterns; we do not ignore them nor do we perpetuate them by engaging with them. We give them support and space without interference so that they are allowed to play out their natural course and dissolve into their background. In this way we begin to see that yoga is a dual process of establishing patterns of practice that allow the possibility of insight to arise. Then, within that insight, we take the opportunity for complete release of the patterns that led to the insight, along with release of the very insight itself. The more complete the release of the patterns, the more we feel liberated on all levels of our being. With the insight we can feel release in our mind and thoughts, just as we feel releasing all through our body—in our navel, in the heart, we are enveloped and penetrated by it.

The next important concept presented in the *Yoga Sūtra* is that of discriminative awareness, or what is called viveka khyātih, and this is one of the keys to full awakening within the *Yoga Sūtra* and within the practice of yoga. Discriminative awareness is also one of the underlying themes of the Sāṁkhya system, upon which the philosophical language of the *Yoga Sūtra* is based. Viveka khyātiḥ is the ability to discriminate or to discern between that which is real and that which is unreal. That which has the qualities of permanence, consciousness, and joy is real;

and those things that are composite, temporary, and unconscious are unreal. The viveka khyātiḥ function of the buddhi continuously sees and disassembles the appearance of false selfhood in whatever is arising as the content of the mind. A good yoga practice helps us to cultivate this capacity for razor-sharp discriminative awareness, and it allows the awareness to manifest through a sense of pure release and nonattachment. In this clear frame of mind, when we are adept at seeing whatever is arising with a sense of discriminative awareness, the state of being called samādhi spontaneously arises. Samādhi is said to be characterized by different layers of deep focus of mind in which the thought process naturally comes together into complete concentration.

Within the *Yoga Sūtra*, Patañjali defines four different layers of samādhi. The first is vitarka, which means the process of deep concentration that is couched in a background of discriminative thinking. When we are in vitarka, it is as if there is an undercurrent of awareness beneath the surface of the concentrated mind—similar to the image of water flowing under a layer of ice. In vitarka there is a mental dialogue of philosophical thought going on; there is movement from thought to counterthought, and then on to other thoughts and new counterthoughts. This forms a metaphorical tube through which the attention flows as it focuses on the actual object being contemplated. In this functioning of mind, a thought can only partially frame an object; it can never quite wrap itself completely around that object, needing a counterthought to cover the angles it missed. This thought process (which is usually in relation to contemplation of gross physical objects or sensations) is like scaffolding that keeps framing the object, forming a background that allows the immediate focus of the mind to be still, clear, and open.

Another deeper level of samādhi is called vicāra, which literally means "inquiry." It is a movement into a chosen, more subtle object. Vicāra might concern those deep, slippery philosophical questions that tend to stun the mind to the point that the questions remain open-ended. It might also be a contemplation of subtle objects, such as the sense fields, rather than particular sense objects. Within vicāra, the backgrounds of things or the fine movements in emotion may even be contemplated.

An even deeper level of samādhi, called ānanda, is that in which the innate character of the mind—which by nature is joy—becomes the very subject of concentration. This joy is considered to be the quality of the open, purified senses themselves without a particular object. Attention to the deep and subtle experiences of the internal yoga body of cleaned-out cakras and nāḍīs also has this quality of innate joy, or ānanda. But remember that this ānanda is not necessarily the joy of the pure ātman; there is still the possible presence of the tamas and rajas guṇas and the operation of egotism in the background.

Deeper still than ānanda is the level of samādhi called asmitā. Asmitā is the principle of I-ness or of I-am-ness, and this level of samādhi deals with the core processes of how the mind generates experience. Asmitā, in addition to being a layer of samādhi, is the principle of mind that can turn into ignorance (avidyā) by superimposing the sense of self onto that which the mind is actually trying to think about. Asmitā is the process of forming the center around which mental maps grow. In samādhi accompanied by asmitā, no maps are forming; only the pure awareness is reflecting into the basic self-making principle, and that principle reflects back, projecting onto the open awareness the sense of "I am."

These four types of concentration are considered to be saṁprajñāta samādhi, that is, samādhi with a seed or samādhi that has some content in the mind. These types of samādhi are different from asaṁprajñāta samādhi, or samādhi without content, which occurs in the gaps that appear when observed content is released or dropped. Within the *Yoga Sūtra*, a mind state with seeds of some gross or subtle structure and a mind state without seeds of thought structure are the two general terms that describe the different forms of samādhi. With this distinction, we realize that the true nature of the mind is to concentrate naturally in samādhi and then to let go into not-knowing. Through the practice of yoga we learn to concentrate in such a way that the mind can take on whatever pattern of sensation, feeling, or thought is present. It is as if the mind were a clear jewel; when placed against any background the jewel reflects and refracts whatever is there without bias. In the same way, a clear mind perceives without breaking the perception into subject and object. In so doing the mind can relax its duties of categorizing, theorizing, and understanding, and it can simply hold the arising form of whatever it perceives as sacred. When *any* particular form of mind is perceived as sacred, it is then released. That release forms the gap in which there is the opportunity to gain true insight and to experience pure awareness—not dependent on a structure and not dependent on a form. Of course, for even the skilled yoga practitioner or meditator, another form appears almost instantly in the mind. The mind then reformulates itself, perhaps on a more subtle or a deeper level. But again, after samādhi forms, that particular new formulation is released. This cycle of the concentration of mind goes deeper and deeper, more and more subtly within the practice of yoga. It is in the gaps—between the forms that arise—that the insight can occur. So samādhi, true and deep concentration of the mind, the ability to really pay attention to what is happening, is the basic tool of yoga. The catch is that the insight of yoga comes only when you are able to release the image on which the mind has concentrated; thus our concept and understanding of samādhi itself must be released so that the practice can continue.

Patañjali defines samādhi as when the object of concentration appears as if empty of self form. This means that the object is a composition of its extended background. It is not separate; it has no ego or self, and it is impermanent. In this way the deeper ego function has nothing to identify with in contemplation. The release of the empty object is natural; it is not a rejection of, or a need to be free of, the object. The "catch and release" cycle of samādhi gives birth to discriminating awareness, which sees the distinction between permanence and impermanence. This awareness gradually causes the reassessment of our whole body, mind, and sense of the world, and it is through discrimination (viveka khyātiḥ) that insight comes within a yoga practice. Knowing this, we can then recognize that samādhi itself is not the goal of yoga; it is instead the primary tool of yoga. As Patañjali points out, if there is identification with the citta vṛtti, with the presentation in the mind, then that is not the state of yoga.

Through yoga we cultivate the ability to take the presentation in the mind and to look at it very, very closely through meditation and eventually through the process of concentrating the mind, through the layering of samādhi. We can experience the insight that there is nobody in the state of mind—our *own* state of mind—there is nobody in the vṛtti. In this way there is no longer identification between the seer and the presentation in the mind, between puruṣa and prakṛti, between pure consciousness and perceptions of mind. Training the mind to rest within this seemingly paradoxical state of insight becomes a practice in and of itself, one that should be approached systematically. It is actually quite simple: whenever there is a presentation in the mind as you are practicing, you simply observe whatever it is that is arising—a feeling, a thought, a sensation. Eventually you are able to take any presentation of mind, and by looking closely you are able to recognize that it is not you. There is nobody there in whatever is presenting itself; there is nobody there in any particular pattern of feeling, thought, or sensation that arises. All of your perceptions are empty of self form. This kind of observation in which the seed patterns of our concentration are released is conducive to the arising of a state of samādhi, and should be practiced through the breath, the body, the sensations, and the mind as continuously as possible. For some rare people the process is quite easy and the release into a state of liberated mind occurs spontaneously. However, most of us do not enter into samādhi without great effort made toward that end.

Samādhi without content, asaṁprajñāta samādhi, could also be called the gap samādhi, suspension samādhi, or residue samādhi. Unless you fall easily into the gap, Patañjali says that the state is preceded by five means: śraddhā, vīrya, smṛti, samādhi, and prajñā. Śraddhā is the practice of faith and trust, which would mean being able to rest and be happy in a state of not-knowing. Vīrya is vigor, as in strength and intensity. The text goes on to say that in order to cultivate trust, one should practice with great vīrya, which means we should practice with great enthusiasm, an enthusiasm that comes by having an open heart during the practice of yoga āsana and prāṇāyāma. So trust and a willingness to sit with and attentively observe whatever is arising as it unfolds, and to be able to rest in the unknown with great vīrya, is at the root of samādhi and the liberation that is attainable through yoga. Smṛti is memory, which allows the perception of long-term patterns and the ability to see many points of view on any topic. Smṛti enables us to learn the lesson of impermanence, and samādhi is the ability to zoom in on anything and to see that it is empty of self form. Prajñā is the discernment and wisdom about the interpenetrating nature of all phenomena that arises from samādhi. It is the clear perception of the ātman in all things.

Patañjali also recommends Īśvara praṇidhāna, surrender to God or to Īśvara, as another means to asaṁprajñāta samādhi. Surrender carries two connotations here. One is that of passive surrender in which the practitioner works to simply let things be as they are—again a sense of trust is foundational to this. In this meaning of Īśvara praṇidhāna, you cease interfering with things as they are arising. You practice this type of surrender within the context of your own body, by ceasing to interfere with your breath, your senses, and then with the whole flow of your mind and emotions. Knowing that all of these are somehow connected to Īśvara, coming from Īśvara, or really *are* Īśvara, you can, with practice, completely accept your actual circumstances. A second interpretation of surrender accepts the possibility of active surrender in which you attend to, offer sacrifice to, and provide service to Īśvara, who is considered to be the original guru or the inner guru in the heart of all beings. Recognizing this primordial relationship makes surrender more palatable for some; it can become quite liberating to actively dedicate the fruits of your actions to Īśvara—and in doing so you are reminded that you are practicing for the benefit of others. Next you render service to Īśvara, which is achieved primarily through the offering of service to others. Patañjali mentions that the word *oṁ* is considered to be the acoustic manifestation of Īśvara, and one possibility for a practice is to chant *oṁ* while reflecting on this as its meaning. Such a practice can release you from a fragmented, externalized mode of thinking. The combination of contemplating the meaning of God or Īśvara and of allowing the sound of *oṁ* to resonate within your body allows you to draw your attention deep into the core of the heart. By attending to Īśvara and by internalizing the essence of the meaning of that act, this type of twofold passive and active surrender is one of the ways of inducing samādhi.

The next section of the *Yoga Sūtra* addresses nine common difficulties and distractions that may arise and interfere within our practice and the manifestation of yoga. How these obstacles manifest at any given time is usually the very key to growth and insight within our own personal practice. It is not really a matter of avoiding the difficulties that resolves them and opens a path to liberation; instead, it is the ability to face the difficulties and the distractions straight on that allows us to truly mature and progress. The first obstacle is vyādhi, which means "disease" or "sickness." This one is easy to understand; of course if you are ill, in pain, or imbalanced, it is very hard to concentrate the mind. So you must deal with illness or disease directly with whatever it takes—going to the doctor, dietary change, lifestyle change, and so on. This is essential if you are to concentrate the mind. Second, we must concentrate and practice as best we can even if we are ill. This usually makes us redefine what practice really is, as we drop back into simple mindfulness of feeling and breath or maybe into prayer. One day we will be sick and we will not get better; we will die. Real practice, attention to the ātman, the real nature of all things, should continue as practice for dying.

The next obstacle to yoga is styāna, meaning "dullness" or "being stuck," and it is also something that must be dealt with if the yoga is to work. In other words, you need vitality. You must not become trapped by tamasic states of mind and body, by imbalanced practices, by lifestyle choices. Yoga āsana, breathing practices, and a waking up of the senses are all helpful in overcoming styāna.

A huge obstacle, one that many people never overcome, is that of saṁśaya or doubt. Doubt is not necessarily a bad thing in and of itself; it simply means that you see two sides to an argument, or that you see two different ways to do a practice. If you cannot decide between the two sides or two perspectives, you are left in a state of confusion and doubt and you may think that since you do not know what to do, you will not do anything at all. This happens all the time in yoga. A student might have two different teachers, and one teacher says to do a yoga pose this way while the other says to do the pose a different way. It puts us in a state of saṁśaya, and we could become paralyzed by that doubt—wondering which teacher is correct, which technique is the safest and most beneficial. The way to overcome saṁśaya, of course, is through śraddhā or trust, by realizing that whatever the different perspectives might be, on a much deeper level they are contingent and depend on context and circumstance. You may not see how they hook together or understand that one is a reaction to the excess of the other, or that one is brilliant and the other is delusional, but with faith and trust, you will not be discouraged or paralyzed. So resolving doubt requires going deeper into the confusion and into the doubt. It means being able to accept the paradox of a situation without contracting so that you can draw your actions out of the very core of your being rather than having to act superficially according to a set belief or a dogma. This is one of the major obstacles to yoga practice, and many, many practitioners give up because of saṁśaya. Generally we cannot accept doubt within ourselves because doubt means to us a betrayal of blind faith and our ego's involvement in our practice, rather than a manifestation of our innate intelligence.

Another obstacle is pramāda, which means "delusion" or "carelessness" and is simply not seeing things as they are. This is the same as the second citta vṛtti (viparaya), and it is overcome by deepening your understanding of the questions at hand; by questioning, consulting others as to their understanding of a subject, studying traditional yoga philosophies, looking deeply within yourself, or by getting feedback from other practitioners. Pramāda is also resolved by paying attention to the feedback from your own body and breath and then responding to that information.

Laziness, or ālasya, is another obstacle to yoga, and it refers to laziness and sloth in the generic sense of not having the energy to do anything. It can also mean an attachment to pleasant states of mind—an attachment to peace, to bliss, or to any pleasant preconception of mind in which we can hide from the realities of existence. This sort of attachment can quickly become a major obstacle because it has a tendency to turn off your inquisitive mind, to sabotage any possibility of exercising discriminative awareness. The attachment of ālasya can cause you to cease pondering the depth of such questions as "What is truth?" A lack of inquisitiveness can cause you to forget that the very nature of the world is suffering, and that it is a place of fragmentation and of death (just as it is a place of bliss). This inability to comprehend impermanence, while hiding in a pocket of dullness or a cloud of intoxication, can lead to more delusion; you can end up missing out not only on yoga but on normal life transformations as well.

The next obstacle is avirati, which means "hankering." Often if you have practiced yoga consistently over some period of time, when you start to settle into the practice, a state of meditation, a calm and clear intensity of feeling deep inside of you, will spontaneously arise. The feeling can be accompanied by a kind of vibrant pleasure, and once it is experienced it is not uncommon to hanker after that feeling or to yearn for it. Sometimes when approaching deep observation or core processes in the body a kind of erotic stimulation begins; the imagination is switched on, and we find ourselves distracted by desires. These pleasurable feelings near the central axis of the body serve as part of the mind's defense mechanism—like a reflex designed to make sure you do not experience the raw intensity and basic real pleasure of the central channel. If you were to experience it, the mind would necessarily have to dissolve into the core of the body, and this could be very dangerous to the ego, so there is a sort of natural repulsion to this intrinsic effect of the practice. Avirati waylays many practitioners who need to learn to observe all types of sensation—pleasant, neutral, and unpleasant—as being merely sensation. The real pleasure, the real rati, is actually right in the central axis in the core of the body. So the closer you get to dissolving into the central axis, the higher the stakes in terms of dissolution of mind into reality. This is why the mind—almost as a defense—tosses out or projects out its own core pleasure as a means of sabotaging its true dissolution.

The next obstacle is bhrānti darśanam, which means a "bad view," a "false vision," or an "erroneous perspective." Essentially it is simply what we might call bad philosophy or taking any philosophical stance to an extreme. Bad philosphy could be a naïve, immature system or, more commonly, a misunderstood system. Good philosophy, cooked in the dialectical fire of time and experience, gives insight, compassion, practical discernment, and joy. In bhrānti darśanam your philosophy becomes more a rigid system in which the depth and context of its ideas are lost. Then the ideas of the system take precedence over life, over the whole, over others—making you unable to appreciate the world or other beings as they are. For example, you may develop a point of view that is so extremely realistic that it becomes too literal, then you cannot see the power of ideas and that there are many ways of thinking about any given situation. Within this literal, almost fundamentalist, mind state, you find yourself grasping at your practice, your religion, and your beliefs too exactly. Alternatively, you can slip into the counterextreme view of this and find yourself becoming a relativist, which causes you to think that all different beliefs and all different practices are the same and equally good. This contemporary form of bhrānti darśanam is the idea of yoga as having no opinions, or that judgment is bad, that "it is all one" in a sort of lackadaisical amorality. With bhrānti darśanam your sense of discrimination (viveka khyāti) or the razor sharpness of mind, is lost.

The next obstacle, alabdha bhūmikatva, is the failure to obtain footing or grounding in any state, and this is a result of an imbalance in the various tensions that compose a yoga practice. For example, there might be a great deal of abhyāsa or practice but no vairāgyam, nonattachment. There might be too much release and no practice at all, or there might be unresolved issues with others or a lack of proper training in meditation or in prāṇāyāma.

The last obstacle is anavasthitatvāni, which literally means "instability." Anavasthitatvāni is when you get your footing, your grounding, through your practice and you start to maintain some continuous focus, but then suddenly the mind jumps away. When you fall into a state of anavasthitatvāni it is usually a result of saṁskāras that are activated by the intensity of a focused mind. Āsana and particularly prāṇāyāma set out to locate and expose these deep trigger points, and the activation of these points makes the mind move away from them. Often instability can be caused by other aspects of your life, besides the yoga practices, which are creating a very deep unconscious agitation. This obstacle is dealt with extensively later in the *Yoga Sūtra* when Patañjali discusses the different limbs of yoga (the aṅgas), and when he underscores the notion that eventually you must carry out the practices of yoga in all aspects of your life in order for yoga to really work.

These obstacles, which are actually forms of distractions of mind, are said to be accompanied by mental and physiological effects described as distress, shaking of the limbs, and agitated breathing. The text offers a very simple solution: if you simply practice one truth—eka tattva—you can eliminate any of the obstacles and their physiological effects. It turns out that eka tattva is the very practice of yoga itself, and it is done by fixing the attention in any one of the elements, any of the sense fields, or any chosen area of concentration. Eka tattva practice is an accepting of everything that is arising, even if it has the appearance of an obstacle, as being the one interconnected reality. Consequently, an honest practitioner will choose as the object of contemplation something that is part of their real-life circumstance. Skilled practitioners will observe that which is in the core of their heart, and they will approach it meditatively and with humility. This is known as the practice of oneness or of one truth. Through the practice of eka tattva you can begin to see that there is depth to whatever it is that appears to be the obstacle. Looking closely at what stands in the way, you can see its complexity and its interpenetration with everything else.

One traditional way of practicing eka tattva is to consider any obstacle as having been placed in your path by the elephant-headed god Gaṇeśa. When you shift your perspectives in this way and are able to imagine a problem that is arising in your life as actually a special gift offered to you by Gaṇeśa himself, then you are more likely to be open to the teaching that lies in the heart of the problem. For example, if you have a headache, you could interpret the pain in your head as not an obstacle, but as the god Gaṇeśa poking you and inviting you to observe the specific sensations and feelings that compose the distraction named "headache." In that way you can begin to enter into a state of meditation in the presence of the obstacle itself. You can even consider the obstacle, its causes, and its effects to be Gaṇeśa himself. With this shift in perspective, the obstacle becomes the object of meditation and is transformed from an obstacle into a gateway into a far deeper level of practice.

Another method for overcoming obstacles is to simply practice friendliness and compassion. The root of so many obstacles has to do with our relationships with others or our relationship with ourselves. Our concepts and beliefs about ourselves and others are a rich source for the creation of obstacles. Patañjali says that if you practice friendliness for those who are happy, if you practice compassion for those who are suffering, if you practice great joy when you meet someone who is full of virtue, and if you practice total indifference when you meet someone who is not virtuous—someone who is creating misery—then the mind will become clear. We have to realize that this is not only an external process, in terms of the people we meet in the world, but that it also has an internal element to it and that it applies to experiencing happiness within our own body and within our own mind—meeting those states within ourselves with this same gesture of equanimity. Practicing friendliness, compassion, joy, and indifference for yourself when you meet these states of being within your own body and mind is a remarkable step toward practicing kindness and compassion toward others as well. This practice is, in a sense, the quick path to yoga because all of the structures and the conditionings of the mind—all of the deep saṁskāra—tie into our heart and into our relationships with others.

Meditating on luminosity or simply contemplating inspiring beings—those who are already enlightened—is another simple and related path toward achieving a liberated mind through yoga. In a sense this is the same as Patañjali's recommendation to practice joy and to experience a deep sense of virtue, and this happens almost automatically when you meet someone who is virtuous. Imagine, for example, one afternoon you are enjoying a cup of tea with friends when into the tea shop walks the Dalai Lama! Even if you were a scoundrel, the mere presence of someone so virtuous would send a shock through you, and you might feel virtuous. Your mind state would shift, your posture would improve, and you would naturally let go of the distractions of mind that had you trapped before he entered the room. Related to this basic idea, Patañjali points out that sometimes even within dreams we have experiences that move us very deeply, affecting us to the extent that a seed for contemplation is planted within us. This, in and of itself, can bring the mind back under control. In fact, this sense of being deeply moved by the virtuous, the real, and the truthful can also happen through meditation on anything that is desirable or agreeable. This is Patañjali's profound teaching: whatever your unique life circumstances are, if you find any kind of pleasing content of the mind that inspires—anything that can actually become a seed for your contemplation—then contemplate it. This teaching from the *Yoga Sūtra* demonstrates a remarkably open-minded approach, composed with the intention of truly teaching people to find whatever method possible to liberate the mind. The *Yoga Sūtra* could even be considered a nonsectarian description of the generic process of cultivating genuine, mystical experience.

There are four books, or pādas, within the *Yoga Sūtra*. As we have seen, the first book, Samādhi Pāda, sets forth the underlying vision of what yoga is and describes the basic techniques of yoga that stabilize that vision. The remaining three pādas describe and deepen this understanding of yoga from slightly different points of view and with different emphasis. The additional pādas allow us to get more comfortable with the basic subject matter of yoga, and they also invite us to explore a little more deeply as we build an understanding of the content that is presented. The second pāda in particular, the Sādhana Pāda, gives us the tools to actually become grounded through the practice of yoga. Most of us have had moments of great inspiration and insight in our lives, but they are usually very brief moments. After an inspirational moment we may suddenly find ourselves back in our ordinary confused and miserable state of consciousness. This is perfectly normal and is a state of affairs that was not foreign to Patañjali. After laying out the basics of yoga in the first pāda he begins to "get real" in the second pāda. In the Sādhana Pāda, Patañjali explores life as it is as the central aspect of the teaching, offering the idea that insights from life can help extend the brief moments of clarity. In this second book an entirely new definition of yoga is offered, that of kriyā yoga, or the yoga of action. Kriyā yoga is defined as having three components; tapas, which means "practice" or "austerity"; svādhyāya, which means "self-study" or "self-reflection"; and Īśvara praṇidhāna, the complete surrender to God or the offering of everything to God.

Tapas is heat; it is the light and the luminosity that arises when we finally set limits for the activities of the mind. Tapas occurs naturally when we enter into a space that we have identified or established sacred. When we enter a mosque or a church, when we are in the presence of a highly intelligent and inspired teacher, or even in a more mundane sense when we step onto our yoga mat, we have set limits for the mind and have defined the space as sacred. Without doing anything, it is likely we will experience a palpable feeling of heat or intensity arising merely through the definition of the space or the situation as exceptional, sacred. Even though there is a natural tendency for tapas to arise, there is also a kind of friction that initially wells up upon entering a new situation or a new space, because the mind (which thrives on distraction) wants to go off and do something else—anything that will not require it to be present and still in an unfamiliar situation. But if we are able to corral the mind when we are entering the space, we begin generating heat, and this happens automatically whenever we concentrate our mind in this way. If we stick with the concentration, then the tapas naturally causes a state of self-reflection through which we begin to inquire into the source of our suffering, so that we can begin to explore and to find out who we really are. From this self-reflection we come to the point of Īśvara praṇidhāna. *Praṇidhāna,* which means "surrender to, or stretch out in front of" can be examined from two different points of view; one passive and the other active. In the context of kriyā yoga, it is helpful to examine the active form in which we offer service to Īśvara who, as was explained earlier, is considered to be the primordial guru within the heart of the yogi. Īśvara is everything: one's intentions; one's actions; the functions of the senses; the flow of the breath; all fantasies, disappointments, emotions. Whatever arises is offered to Īśvara . Essentially through this offering to Īśvara we cultivate the vision that Īśvara is in the core of the heart of all other beings, including all other human beings. We discover that Īśvara is actually their ultimate identity. By rendering service to others in this way, first through having the vision of who they truly are and then by attending to them as if they were God, we can quickly gain access to the innermost depths of yoga.

One purpose of kriyā yoga is to bring about samādhi. In this deep meditative state, in which we participate fully with whatever the object of awareness is, there is no sense of subject or object, and the state of samādhi itself becomes our basic tool for probing into the depths of reality. Another purpose of kriyā yoga is to lessen the kleśas, which are the torments or the afflictions that are considered to be the root of suffering. There are five kleśas mentioned in the *Yoga Sūtra*. Four of them grow out of the first, which is avidyā, or ignorance. Ignorance is said to be the confusion of that which is temporary, unclean, impermanent—that which is not really the ātman or the self—with that which is permanent, pure, and happy. This basic misidentification of the temporary as the permanent, of the happy as the unhappy, of the pure as the impure, this confusion generates all sorts of miseries. The second misery is asmitā, which means "I am-ness" or the establishment of a sense of self as separate from all else. When you see yourself as separate, the mind goes in search of objects that will satisfy the senses, needing to accumulate all kinds of things in order to prove its own false hypothesis that it is something that is quite unique and separate from everything else. From this confused state, rāga, or desire, appears, accompanied by a sense of grasping for those things that will support the false hypothesis that the self is separate. This is also accompanied by dveṣa, which is a state of repulsion or rejection of those things that are perceived as being threatening or of no use to the falsely defined separate self. A fundamental truth quite difficult for the mind to comprehend is that when we are grasping or holding on to something, we are also pushing away its opposite with an equal intensity. This process of grasping and rejecting is a root cause of great misery. This is because the things that are being sought are actually incapable of giving us the type of dissolution and pleasure that the mind is actually searching for. The quest for and attainment of objects is ultimately an inadequate method of returning the mind to its natural state of samādhi—which is ultimately what allows for true pleasure and lasting happiness.

The first part of the Sādhana Pāda offers a real vision of heaven and hell, which can be imagined as a gigantic tree whose roots of suffering, of hatred, or of hell, grow and are firmly rooted into the earth. As deep as these roots extend down, the branches and the leaves of its opposite, or of heaven, reach up. But the tree is just one thing, a single aspect of a much bigger matrix of interconnected expressions of life. If we contemplate the image of the tree, we eventually realize that all of its parts are composed of the primordial constituents of prakṛti, of creative energy. We can then let go of the image of the whole tree, knowing that, even in its complexity, it is not separate from its background, and in that release we can begin the process of yoga. When we have insight into the complete creation of our mind and a new vision of the entire world as being one large interconnected web of happiness and distress, heat and cold, of innumerable sets of opposites, we come to the final kleśa, one final root of suffering. It is said that even wise people suffer from this kleśa, abhiniveśa, which means "clinging to life." Interestingly enough, abhiniveśa, or the fear of death, is intimately connected to the deeper experiences of a mature yoga practice in which we start to feel that everything is dissolving around us as if we were dying. Not only are things we would like to have dissolve dispersing, but we see all things, even those we do not want to be rid of, also disappearing. We recognize that things both way out in the world and those close at hand are melting away, as are things deep inside the very core of our own mind—within our emotions and our own bodies. The initial reaction to this recognition of our own impermanence is naturally one of ultimate fear or panic. Yet if we can simply rest with the knowledge that all is impermanent, and if we can trust in the process of not-knowing—both are qualities integral to change—then insight into the truth of impermanence is possible. Understanding this is considered to be the dawning of the light of discriminative knowledge. This sense that everything around us is composed merely of vibration and is therefore impermanent is a profound insight of a good yoga practice, and it reveals how out of the field of avidyā, the ignorance of not realizing that everything is impermanent, the other kleśas easily grow. The real work of yoga, therefore, is to remove the ignorance from which this sense of separateness stems.

It is said that the kleśas can be either manifest—that we are aware of the confusion and pain they cause and the sense of separateness and ego, grasping, revulsion, or fear we may feel—or that they may be nonmanifest, experienced as emotions or discomfort we do not clearly identify with a root cause. Kleśas that in the subtle form, lying deep within the core of the mind, can be shifted by what is called pratiprasava, which means to "reverse the flow," to turn the current of the kleśas back on themselves. For instance, if we become angry or distraught for no apparent reason, we may still notice and identify this sign of discomfort we call "anger." If at that point we can release the wave of emotion that is sweeping over us, we may realize that the way we feel might be connected to the recent death of a friend, or even our subconscious awareness of the concept of death due to the news of a public figure passing away; it could also be related to an underlying discomfort with anything that has changed or transformed within our world. We can then trace our emotions, fears, and attachments back through our primordial repulsion to death and impermanence, our attachment to the one who has died or to the situation that has shifted, and our identification with our concept of ourselves through them. Eventually our distress can be traced back to the fact that deep within us there is a part that feels completely separate and isolated from all else—the underlying cause of our suffering, which is the ignorance known as avidyā. Having traced the charged feelings and our mental constructs back to this original source within our minds, and having seen the empty nature of our misperception of separateness, we can then allow that train of consciousness to dissolve back into our hearts and minds, bringing awareness back into the circumstances that are arising in the here and now. We may notice the flow of the kleśas at any point, from avidyā through asmitā to abhiniveśa. Placing attention on the vṛtti pattern, we trace the vṛtti back through the flow of the kleśas, resolving the suffering we are experiencing back through ego into fundamental ignorance. Those kleśas that have manifested as citta vṛttis, those aspects of our suffering we more easily name, such as the anger we may feel when our ego is challenged or the frustration that arises when we cannot get something we are attached to having, these more blatant kleśas can be dissolved by practicing dhyāna or meditation on the immediate mind state that is arising. So again we see that the entire practice of yoga, the path to liberation in fact, is to get to the root of whatever is presenting itself.

This process of bringing awareness into the deep and underlying concept of separateness that keeps us stuck in the realm of mind and emotion is not an easy task. It is one that must be approached again and again and again as the mind quite naturally slips back toward the secure realm of ego function, of identifying us as separate from others and the rest of the world. Until we actually take up yoga, we tend to spend our time and arrange our activities with a focus on trying to repair the surface of things in order to create a state of happiness and pleasure in our lives. As we go through life and countless experiments within our own experience of the world, as we experience trials within our work and our relationships with others, we discover that just smoothing things out on the surface does not really work; this never results in lasting happiness. As long as the root of suffering and the deep conditioning that is held within the memory is still there, all of the habits and techniques of avoidance that we have developed to help us navigate through life (perhaps through many, many lifetimes) will not actually eliminate our suffering. This is because the cause of our suffering is the great ignorance of avidyā—the misperception that we are separate from our background. Of course this is complicated by the fact that it is the same confusion that automatically leads us to attempt to repair the surface of our lives. The insight that we are not separate, that truth or God is the interpenetrating link that lies within each "separate" being, is the starting point on a path of liberation from the suffering caused by avidyā. When we begin to see that each molecule, each thought, feeling, or sensation is part of an interconnected web of life, we necessarily develop the skill of discriminative awareness that enables us to function with clarity and compassion.

In this light, the *Yoga Sūtra* describes eight different limbs with which to cultivate discriminative knowledge. If you consider the idea of pure insight, you might think that *one* limb would be the true practice since the insight is one immediate experience of truth. However, even though it is insight that gives us knowledge, it is not a practice in and of itself. The only way to truly attain yoga is to have many limbs, or to approach the teaching from multiple angles and to cultivate the insight from various aspects of awareness. Trying to pedal down a path on a unicycle is very challenging especially if you come to an obstacle. Easier than a unicycle is a bicycle, easier than a bicycle, a tricycle because you have lateral stability, and so on. So it is with the study of a complex subject such as yoga; approaching it through only one perspective or studying only one limb is far more difficult than taking a multifaceted approach. The *Yoga Sūtra* describes a vehicle for insight that has eight limbs, something like a spider. So when we come to an obstacle in yoga we are able to approach it from many different points of view —from its physiological angles, its psychological viewpoints, and its philosophical perspectives. The different limbs of yoga allow us to consider the problem of existence and to cultivate a sense of insight into truth in a diverse, comprehensive, and grounded way. This eight-limbed vehicle of a balanced yoga practice is called aṣṭāṅga yoga. *Aṣṭa* means "eight," *aṅga* means "limbs." The eight limbs are: yama, ethical practice; niyama, observances; āsana, postures; prāṇāyāma, extension of the internal breath; pratyāhāra, abstraction of the senses; dhāraṇā, concentration; dhyāna, meditation; and samādhi, deep meditation in which all sense of a subject and an object disappear. These eight limbs at first appear to be sequential, as if you must begin with the yamas and work your way systematically through the others before having a brush with the liberated and compassionate feelings associated with samādhi. Upon closer examination we discover that the limbs of the practice are intertwined; they are each contained within one another and the practice of each limb, just as the experience of samādhi itself is forever deepening as we continue to practice.

Even though all good yoga practices must stem from a strong ethical foundation (the yamas and niyamas), many people begin their study of yoga with an āsana practice. Āsana is comprehensible and is not as intimidating as the other limbs because it involves moving the body, twisting it into all sorts of interesting shapes, and dropping into the feelings and sensations that arise as the body is worked. For many beginners it is sensible to introduce the practice through the postures. After some time practicing āsana we are likely to become interested in meditation or the idea of ethical relationships may pique our interest, until eventually we see the connection between the various limbs of the practice. Students often find that they need to emphasize different limbs at different times as their practice evolves and their study deepens. As we become more advanced in the practice, we begin to realize that none of the limbs are the actual "goal" of yoga: how long we can hold the breath in prāṇāyāma, whether or not we can put our leg behind our head while practicing āsana, or how quickly we can focus the mind, is not what matters. The "goal" (if you could call it such) is to reach a state of discriminative insight, to have a direct experience of the nature of pure consciousness and pure being, as well as to have an experience of the fundamental character and form of the mind itself.

In addition to the limbs of study within a yoga practice, the *Yoga Sūtra* also describes five yamas, or foundations of ethical behavior, that are essential for a yoga practice. Other traditional texts mention ten yamas, some even mention fifteen, but we can get the basic idea from these five; behaving toward ourselves and others in a clear and ethical manner is at the root of the practice. The first yama is nonviolence, or ahiṁsā. This simply means to do no harm, to cause no suffering either to others or to one's self. We find that ahiṁsā is not so much something that requires effort and will, but rather that it flows naturally out of a consistent yoga practice. As we progress in the practice of āsana and prāṇāyāma, our powers of attentiveness and observation increase and we start to notice how our own attitudes of rāga and dveṣa, our feelings of attraction and repulsion, are spontaneously activated even to our own sense fields and to our own breath. By practicing nonviolence toward ourselves we automatically start to respect even our immediate sense perceptions as sacred. In the presence of anything we find sacred it is quite natural to feel kind, loving, compassionate, and connected. So nonviolence is the very first yama of the beginning stage of the eight-limbed yoga practice, and it is profoundly important.

The yama that Patañjali discusses as following nonviolence is satya, or truthfulness. This simply means to speak what is true and honest, and then to act in accordance with that. Satya does not necessarily mean factual truth, but it means to act in accordance with the truth of the *Yoga Sūtra,* which is the truth of pure consciousness liberated in the present moment. People who fancy themselves to be exceedingly truthful, and who are perhaps even a little bit self-righteous, will sometimes use factual truth in ways that actually violate the vow of ahiṁsā or nonviolence; they may use facts in ways that breach the deeper principles of truth and nonviolence. For example, it could be factually true that someone has a very ugly nose, but simply pointing that out to them and to others would serve no purpose other than to humiliate and embarrass the person. Satya, therefore, is not established as the first of the yamas; instead it follows and builds upon ahiṁsā, which is the principle of nonharming and kindness.

The third yama, asteya, means to "not steal." Of course this applies on the most obvious level and means to not be a thief, to not rob banks or the grocery store, to not steal bicycles and cars. But asteya also implies many more subtle levels of not-stealing, such as not plagiarizing ideas without giving credit for them. It means not accumulating for yourself things that do not really belong to you, not being a phony, not holding on to things that ultimately are not yours. It even applies to things that come into the sphere of our influence, for example, physical property—a house we might own—which must ultimately be seen as impermanent like all else. In the end, asteya means to not claim anything as being exclusively ours and separate from all else. It could even be considered a form of stealing if we cannot see that our very body and our sense perceptions are not ours, that they are not to be separate from their background, the interlinking web of existence of the life we are part of. When practicing asteya we see things as part of an interconnected whole, and with that insight, we can release everything to be just as it is so that all may flow in its natural and true way.

The next yama, brahmacarya, is often translated as "celibacy." It is helpful to understand the literal meaning of brahmacarya as well, which is to "act in Brahman" or to "act in God" or "pure consciousness." Ultimately brahmacarya implies a highly ethical sexual practice. This could mean you are leading a monastic life, or if you are involved in a sexual relationship, brahmacarya would mean that the relationship is one that follows ahiṁsā, satya, and asteya; the first of the yamas in which we do no harm to others through our relationship and we do not lose our vision that deep in his or her heart the other is the ātman. Brahmacarya can actually mean, in an esoteric sense, one who enters into what is called the brahma nāḍī, which is the channel within the central axis of the body. Brahma nāḍī is said to be a thin thread that is visualized within the suṣumnā nāḍī (the central channel) and once the prāṇa enters into the brahma nāḍī, one tastes or has a direct experience of reality. So to be a true brahmacarya does not mean someone who egotistically denies themselves the pleasures of life, but it means one who has entered into the very heart of reality.

The last of the yamas presented in the *Yoga Sūtra* is aparigraha, which means to "not grasp at things." Aparigraha is the tendency of the mind, under the sway of the ego, to simply snatch at things and claim them to be its own. The mind moves about as if saying, "This, I identify with, that, I do not." The mind quite naturally does this in all spheres of activity—the political, economic, interpersonal, psychological realms, even in our private thoughts we can start to collect and accumulate things. All of this grasping becomes a huge encumbrance and an obstacle that interferes in our relationships with other beings. It is a major obstacle to a deep yoga practice since relationship is at the core of the practice, and the quintessence of relationship is trust, fairness, and love. If the yamas are practiced, then love is allowed to flow freely and to function right at the center of our lives. The practice of the yamas as described in the *Yoga Sūtra* is considered to be the mahāvrata, or the great vow, and it means that for anyone engaged in the discipline of yoga, the yamas are practiced under all circumstances and at all times. With this deeper understanding of what yoga truly is, we find that we practice yoga all day, every day.

The yamas are followed in the *Yoga Sūtra* by a description of the niyamas, which are specific yogic disciplines. The first niyama, śauca,or cleanliness, has several layers of meaning. The immediate meaning is that of personal hygiene, which is, of course, vital to a good yoga practice because it relates to the prevention of disease and unnecessary sickness. But to be clean also means to have your senses refreshed and vibrant as a means of facilitating the observation of things clearly and as they truly are. It is kind of like keeping the windshield of your car clean, which really does help when driving. So keeping not only the body clean but maintaining the environment that we live in a very simple and clean manner is conducive to being able to sit down and practice yoga. Śauca makes it easy to practice the next of the niyamas, which is saṅtoṣa, contentment. Contentment is the ability to be happy right now for no particular reason at all. You can actually cultivate this feeling by simply deciding, "Right now I am going to be content." This may sound overly simplistic, but what it actually means is that right now you are going to temporarily suspend your worries, your cares and desires, and you are going to drop your theories and conclusions about what is happening and simply experience the radiance of pure being as it is. The ability to be content with life's circumstances, the skill of seeing the sacred nature of the world as it is arising and of being patient as the world discloses itself, is a profoundly deep capacity that we cultivate, and it is also one of the keys to the entire practice of yoga. This does not mean that you have to agree with everything that arises, nor does it mean that you should see everything as perfect and wonderful, or that you disengage from your responsibilities in life. Instead it means that you are present with the raw truth—good, bad, ugly, smelly, or sublime—of whatever is arising. It means that you cultivate a clear and compassionate space within which life unfolds, and that your actions reflect this clarity and compassion. From a state of contentment we can then practice tapas or practices that generate the heat of yoga. With the clarity that results from tapas we can then go deep inside and practice svādhyāya, which is self-reflection or meditation on the self. Through this flow of the practice we are able to surrender to Īśvara, to have trust and to give all to God. Through this, samādhi is achieved, and through samādhi we go back deep into the very root of the mind, and eventually we become fully grounded in the present moment, grounded in discriminative awareness.

The next of the limbs and probably the most famous limb in the eight-wheel-drive vehicle of yoga is āsana or postures. Although most Westerners see the postures as the main part of what is considered to be a yoga practice, there are only two verses in the *Yoga Sūtra* that deal with posture. Stepping back from our own preconceptions, we should reevaluate what yoga āsana might actually be. According to the *Tejo*

Bindu Upaniṣad, a good yoga āsana is that from which meditation can arise easily and spontaneously. Contrary to the way some of us sometimes approach āsana practice, it is not a way of torturing the body. The word āsana comes from the verbal root *as*, meaning "to sit"; so in some contexts *āsana* simply means a good seat, a nice chair, or a comfortable cushion. Through the practice of āsana the body itself is transformed into a seat, and it simply rests in that pleasant place. Yoga becomes the platform from which pure awareness is allowed to arise. A good posture is considered to be one that is sthira and sukha, sthira meaning "grounded" or "stable," and sukha meaning "happy" or "easy." Within an āsana practice, once we are grounded and happy in a posture, we then come to the point where all effort within the posture ceases and the mind naturally goes into contemplation of ananta, or a reflection on infinity. Of course within the realm of the yoga matrix, wherever the mind happens to rest, whatever the immediate presentation of the mind is, *that* is experienced as infinity, as endless and interconnected. It is through the practice of yoga āsana that most of us can actually experience this infinite quality of even the most ordinary everyday experience. When the yoga poses are established well, then the practitioner is ready for the beginning of the next limb of the practice, prāṇāyāma.

- When first studying prāṇāyāma (the breathing practices associated with yoga), we should remember the axiom within the yoga tradition that the mind, the citta, always moves in relation to the inner breath or the prāṇa. As such, prāṇāyāma is the practice of stretching or removing the restrictions on the prāṇa, and in a sense, it is a way to create freedom or a release of the inner breath. Prāṇāyāma is often mistranslated as the "practice of controlling the prāṇa." However, the word *ayāma* literally means "to remove the controls or the restrictions," so prāṇāyāma is more accurately translated as "taking away the restrictions that inhibit the deep and natural flow of the breath." Prāṇāyāma practices initially train us to focus on and to cultivate a conscious flow of the prāṇa through what superficially appear to be techniques of controlling the breath, but the practice is never one of inhibiting the breath. Instead, in prāṇāyāma practice we travel deep into the core of the body and likewise into the core of the mind, and through the breath we start to decondition the mind by unraveling some of the associations that have been made within the mind (and therefore within the emotions and physical body as well) over the years. We observe and allow thoughts and sensations that we may experience deep in our guts to untangle. The practice of prāṇāyāma is said to remove the obscuration of the light, and this makes the next form of the practice, meditation, very easy.

It is said that the first four limbs—yamas, niyamas, āsana, and prāṇāyāma—are the external limbs. These are the things you can really sink your teeth into and actually *do*. You can work with these first four limbs, you can wrestle with them, and if you get these outer forms of the practice very clear and strong, then the inner contemplative limbs become far easier to approach. The contemplative limbs are: pratyāhāra, which is sense withdrawal; dhāraṇā, or concentration of the mind; dhyāna, which is meditation; and samādhi. As you practice you will notice that these inner limbs are very difficult, virtually impossible, to even approach if the outer limbs are not established clearly. For example, if you sit down to meditate and your ethical life is in upheaval, if your emotional life is confused and your body is misaligned, or if your breath is erratic, then it is going to be nearly impossible to rest in a state of meditation and to observe the agitations of mind clearly. Working with the first four external limbs of the practice reduces the likelihood of these sorts of outer turmoil in your life because you will have become more balanced, and consequently the inner limbs of the practice will be far more accessible. It is important to note too that the meditative aspects of a yoga practice can also become distractions if they are practiced from a place of ego. Within the *Yoga Sūtra,* Patañjali describes the means to making meditation practice true and grounded as being contingent not only on being stable in the first four limbs of the practice, but also as being dependent on the practitioner's ability to distinguish between what is being experienced as the object of consciousness and consciousness.

As we examine the different aṅgas or limbs of yoga, we tend to move through them in a sequential progression in order to understand them clearly. In practice, however, just as we experienced the kleśas, we must constantly loop back through all the limbs if we are to remain clear and grounded. In prāṇāyāma, for example, we have to go back to the yamas, to the niyamas, and to āsana. So the practice is always starting over, always feeding back in on itself. In the sequence of the aṅgas presented in the *Yoga Sūtra,* pratyāhāra follows prāṇāyāma. Pratyāhāra literally means "to not eat, to not consume." When we experience something through any of our senses, there is a natural tendency to grasp whatever it is. In that grasping, the mind tends to superimpose a name or a concept onto the raw sensations associated with the experience—it is as if we are eating and digesting it. This is a natural process of the mind, which needs some kind of referential knowledge in order to make sense of any experience. If it is not consuming the sense objects, then the mind is usually pushing the sense objects away with the same type and intensity of fragmenting energy. Pratyāhāra, therefore, is the release of the urge to gobble up what comes into our senses, to leave the sense fields and allow them to be just as they are. In a healthy yoga practice, with this release the senses are then free to follow the mind, which allows the mind to spontaneously move into meditation. Just as bees will follow the queen bee, so the indriyas, the senses, will follow the mind to a deeper yoga practice when they are set free from the consumption of conceptually generated objects. In pratyāhāra the sense objects themselves are released; they are not rejected nor are they grasped, but instead they are appreciated as pure vibration rather than objects. It is said that the perfection of pratyāhāra is to see or to directly experience the ātman or pure being through any or all of the senses.

Following pratyāhāra is the sixth limb, dhāraṇā, which is defined as tying the mind to one field of experience. Keeping the mind within the activities of one aspect of awareness might seem to insinuate that this type of concentration has an exclusive nature to it, that there is some sort of effort or decision that "wills" us to focus the mind as if with blinders. But concentration actually happens spontaneously—through the practice of releasing the mind into the full field of awareness rather than attempting to block off any of the aspects of the field of perception that are naturally arising. Dhāraṇā can happen through a practice, but it also happens under normal circumstances; everybody does it whether or not they practice yoga. When you encounter a subject that is of great interest to you and you start to focus on it, you are "tying your mind to the field of one experience." You block out all other areas of potential awareness in order to concentrate and satisfy your mind. For example, you hear something interesting, or you come across something in nature, or you see something on TV that catches your attention. If it is particularly noteworthy, you naturally sharpen your focus toward whatever you are experiencing. You allow the mind to concentrate fully by settling the distractions of mind and also through how you use your breath and whatever subtle and gross movements you make with your body. Of course eventually you may experience some conflict as there are other aspects of your mind that are not being allowed into the center ring. You will notice that there are always pressures from within and without that are vying for your mind's attention; however, in order to concentrate, your mind temporarily seals itself off from this other input.

As the yoga deepens we find that dhāraṇā (concentration) progresses into the next of the eight limbs, which is dhyāna, or meditation. Within this state of being there is a flow of the mind into only one field of awareness, and this causes a spontaneous sense of relaxation and release. In dhyāna there is no longer the heat of conflict between fragmented aspects of mind, and at the same time there is an appreciation for the fact that whatever is within the field of awareness possesses a truly sacred quality. Sacred, in this context, simply means an unknown, a mysterious, or a captivating quality that invites the mind to flow easily. In this state of mind, the background—or those things that lie outside the chosen field of awareness—is intuited to be interconnected with what is within the foreground—those things that lie within the field of awareness. Background and foreground may be appreciated as distinctly different when we are in a state of dhyāna, but they are not seen as actually separate. Psychologically, there is a sense that the mind does not really have to move in order to be concentrated. Then, as the meditation deepens, there comes a point at which the mind dissolves into the present experience, and there is no longer any sense of a subject and an object, there is no observer looking at an observed. Instead, the chosen field or the chosen object of contemplation appears to be empty of any mentally constructed separate existence. At this point the chosen field of contemplation is seen to be empty of a svarūpa, empty of its own self form, and this is considered to be samādhi.

The last three limbs of the eight-limbed path—dhāraṇā, dhyāna, and samādhi—are collectively called saṁyama, which means "to draw together," and these three things taken together as saṁyama are considered to be a primary tool of yoga. Through saṁyama we are able to go back to the beginning of practice in order to examine the body in the context of an interconnected pattern of existence that goes infinitely beyond the boundaries of the body itself. We are able to take the yoga āsanas into unbelievable realms of subtlety, getting in touch with remarkably deep aspects of the sensation and feeling that arise as a means of allowing us to access profoundly subtle aspects of the mind. Through the same saṁyama, a mature prāṇāyāma practice is developed, and it is also through saṁyama that we start to understand relationships; we begin to understand other beings. All eight limbs of yoga are made increasingly functional and useful once we get into the last three, which, more immediately than the other limbs, help us to develop the ability to pay attention to what is actually happening right here, right now.

Ultimately, through this progression of practice and understanding, we have insight into the interconnectedness of the mind and the universe. We can experience everything as being within a matrix in which any chosen point of sensation or perception contains all of the other potential points of sensation or perception exposing the natural self-luminous quality of being as it manifests. We can see then that yoga practice is simply an unfolding of the mind using a series of practices that allow us to pay very close attention. As our practice ripens, our heart becomes vast and more sensitive, and at the same time our intelligence becomes keener. We simultaneously develop discriminating intelligence, which allows us to go deeper and deeper until the fundamental urges of the three guṇas (rajas, tamas, and sattva) no longer have an object toward which they project. Prakṛti's three guṇas are then said to have fulfilled their real purpose, which is to reveal puruṣa through discriminating awareness. At this stage of practice, whenever an object arises we are able to see right through it as being empty of self. Without the prop of false selfhood to support them, the three guṇas fall out of our perceptual presence back into the primordial ground of creative energy. At this point the falling away of the most subtle and deep aspects of the creative mind reveals, once and for all, the true nature of the self or of the ātman. This complete unfolding of the mirror of prakṛti is the conclusion of the *Yoga Sūtra* and is called kaivalya, or "aloneness," which is seen to be the ecstatic and essential nature of all beings. It is important to note that in this context you are not alone in your aloneness. What is meant by kaivalya is that we are alone from prakṛti; we are not entangled in and caught up in the strands of our own creative energy, an energy that functions through the principle of overlap and superimposition. We are not engaged in the energy and mind states that create time and space and multiple universes, we are not ruled by the structure of separateness from which the mind creates suffering. So the *Yoga Sūtra* gives us a radical vision of the potential of our own lives. The *Yoga Sūtra* is like a potent medicine, one that cures us of our avidyā by waking us up into our open, fresh, radiant nature. It is good to take little sips of the medicine now and then, and occasionally it is even a good idea to take a big swig of it. The teachings of the *Yoga Sūtra* will always remind us of the true depths of the great variety of practices and the true potential of our own lives. Otherwise it is very easy to oversimplify, to lose sight of the subtlety, the nuance, the complexity, and the beauty of what yoga actually is.

9

Cutting Through Fundamentalism

I bow to the two lotus feet of the
(plurality of) Gurus, which awaken insight
into the happiness of pure Being, which are
the complete absorbtion into joy,
the jungle physician, eliminating the delusion
caused by the poison of saṁsāra (conditioned existence).

I prostrate before the sage Patañjali who has thousands of radiant,
white heads (as the divine serpent, Ananta) and who has, as far
as his arms, assumed a human form, holding
a conch shell (divine sound),
a wheel (a discus of light or time) and a sword (discrimination).
OṀ

THE EPIGRAPH ABOVE is a traditional invocation for aṣṭāṅga yoga, which is often chanted before beginning a yoga practice. It is a meditation on the guru, or the teacher, and in particular to Patañjali who, as the presumed author of the *Yoga Sūtra*, is an important guru to all who study yoga. This idea of a guru is possibly one of the most exotic and, at the same time, problematic aspects of a traditional yoga practice for everyone. Part of the problem is that the term *guru* has been co-opted in modern culture, and many people have all sorts of peculiar associations with it. If we can understand the function of the teacher or the guru within the context of traditional yoga, we can step clear of some of the problems and potential entanglements that having or rejecting a teacher might bring to mind. As is traditionally true for most subjects that are deep and at points paradoxical, it is through a guru that you learn yoga. In any complex discipline, it is incredibly helpful to find someone as a teacher who has progressed within thc field, even if she or he have not mastered it, so that when doubts, questions, and conflicts arise (as they should and are bound to) you have a source that can offer you a learned perspective and assistance in understanding. In terms of yoga, having a teacher is doubly important because not only can the guru shed light on areas of confusion, but the relationship itself becomes a demonstration of a fundamental building block in the ethical and theoretical web of the philosophy itself—that clear and strong relationships are built on the ability to discover a connection to the interpenetrating nature of pure consciousness. The particular beliefs and techniques, the specifics of the art a guru transmits in yoga, are secondary to the essential love and relationship that are established in the present moment between student and teacher.

The word *guru* has a number of meanings. Probably the most common is that the guru is the "remover of darkness." This translation is particularly appropriate within the context of yoga in that the darkness of ignorance is removed right from the core of your heart simply by your relationship to your teacher, through the realization of the type of love and deep respect that one might have with a teacher. The word *guru* also means "heavy." Of course this does not mean that the teacher must eat immense quantities of food and become spherical (though some have, and they have helped to form one of the more endearing images we often have of the guru). Gurus are considered heavy in the sense that they are not moved, nor are they uprooted in their understanding, by others. Good teachers are not swayed by the changing phenomena of the world; they are able to rest completely silent and serene at the center of their own experience. An interesting counter to the idea of the guru being "heavy" is that within the guru-student relationship, the disciple is called laghu, which means "featherweight." This of course insinuates that the student is not filled with the same depth of knowledge as the

disciple . laghu . light - featherweight

teacher, and for this reason it is not uncommon that students beginning their studies often find themselves orbiting around the teacher almost as if attracted, for better or for worse, by the immense gravitational field of the guru. Eventually, by sticking with the studies and by embodying the teachings, the laghu becomes guru—the student finds the phenomenon of the guru right in the core of his or her own heart. At the same time, established and true gurus will rarely identify their egos directly with the principle that is discovered by their students, that principle which lies deep in their cores. So if someone claims to be a guru, if they assert that they are the light of true awakening and enlightenment, this should raise a red flag in any student's mind. Ego absorption is the unfortunate root of a big problem that arises for many gurus who stray from their own path as a teacher by becoming so enamored by their greatness, as projected through the eyes of their students, that they themselves fall prey to the delusion of their own grandeur.

The first part of the aṣṭāṅga yoga invocation that appears as the epigraph to this chapter makes reference to the two feet of the guru, which reveal the paradoxical nature of all relationships, which, by definition, are two or more entities meeting. Like the two feet of the guru, there are at least two perspectives brought to every relationship—and therefore the potential for paradox is always present whenever alternative perspectives are pulled out of their mutual background and seen as separate. The invocation, with reference to the two feet or multiplicity of perspectives, sets the stage for the fact that insight is most easily drawn from binocular vision. Often when we relate to another person we do so from only one perspective, formed out of our preconceptions of who we are, what we need, what we want, juxtaposed with who we imagine that other person to be, what we envision them being able to do for us, or what we imagine they can do in relation to our sense of our self. This invariably causes problems.

The teacher is said to have a red foot and a white foot, symbolizing that the two feet of the guru allow light from different perspectives to shine on the teaching. Within many yoga traditions these two feet are visualized as resting in the crown of the head. The white foot represents metaphorical teaching, meaning that the teachings of the guru are not to be taken literally and should be seen to have a deeper purpose than the specific metaphor that conveys their meaning. The red foot represents the literal teaching, through which the guru teaches how to deal with immediate and practical circumstances in the world. A complete relationship with a teacher is very deep and spiritual and at the same time extraordinarily immediate and practical because two forms of knowledge are being brought to light simultaneously. In the best of teachings, esoteric or mystical knowledge is interpenetrated by knowledge about the practical arts of life—how to eat intelligently, how to interact with others compassionately, how to go about doing what needs to be done in the world skillfully. There is an art to seeing those practical aspects in context, and it requires an even greater amount of expertise to release the practical understanding and intelligence in order to connect to the more esoteric side of life—dissolving into the depths of the immediate relationship with the subject matter, the teacher, and the present moment.

The guru of gurus is said to be the real teacher, but rather than identifying the gurus' guru as some particular or composite person or a

Two Feet (7)

The two feet of the guru represent a dialectical process that dissolves the ignorance of the single perspective. The feet symbolize the traditional sets of opposites such as Śiva and Śakti, sun and moon, prāṇa and apāna, iḍā and piṅ galā, night and day, pluralism and absolutism, relativism and fundamentalism, monism and dualism, insight and skillful means, emptiness and compassion, male and female. One foot is in the realm of metaphor and myth. The other is grounded in the real, everyday world of blood and bones. In teachings of non-dualism, truth is presented in two ways: as the supreme, absolute truth and then the truth of the practical, relative world. The two feet of the guru allow you to live in a realm in which no formula or doctrine is absolute, and a realm in which you have to take a practical stand in order to deal with practical matters. Paramārtha, or the supreme truth, is said to be the truth that all is Brahman. Saṁvṛti is the truth that conceals this ultimate reality (that all is Brahman) and makes us take a stand and act decisively in the everyday world.

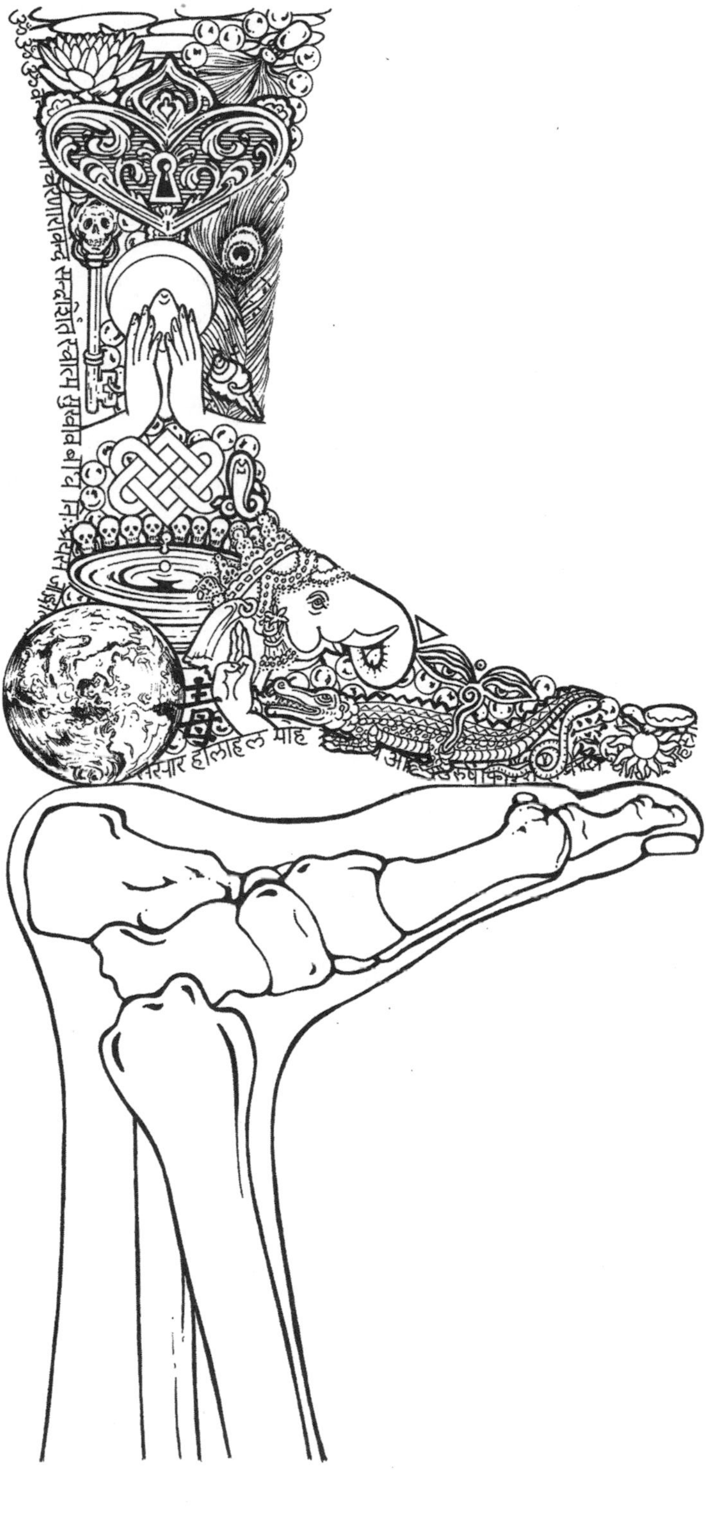

specific formula, it is better to simply set aside the inquiry as to who the teacher of the teachers actually is. In fact, it is essentially the mind's ability to rest in the unknown that reveals the true teacher of teachers, and in one sense this ability *is* the gurus' guru. This kind of open and trusting mind, accompanied by constant inquiry, is essential to the yogic tradition, within which all conclusions we may arrive at are subject to further questioning. The inquiring heart takes all conclusions and looks so closely at them that ultimately we have to release them all. This infinite fascination with knowledge is therefore what we seek in a relationship with the guru, or in fact with any teacher and with all of the presentations of life itself. Through a healthy relationship with a teacher we have insight into the fact that keeping the heart open and of allowing inquiry to flow is at the root of all relationships. With any being to whom you become intimately close, the relationship is always an open question.

An unlocked heart is one that is looking so sincerely and so deeply that all of the multiplicity of answers that arise as thought and form are allowed to dissolve within the intensity of the inquiry. Meditating on the two feet of the guru (the paradoxical nature of all relationships) dispels what is called the saṁsāra hālāhala. In Indian mythology hālāhala is said to be the poison that arose when the gods and the demons joined forces in a yogic process of churning the ocean of saṁsāra (conditioned existence) in the attempt to produce the nectar of immortality. According to the myth, the first product that arose from their churning was not the nectar immortality, but something called hālāhala, which was a deadly toxic by-product of the yogic process. As it arose and washed up on the beaches around this yogic ocean, all sentient beings began feeling the ill effects of the toxin. Not knowing what to do to get rid of this poisonous substance, so the myth goes, they called upon the great god Śiva. (Śiva, by the way, is considered to be the guru of gurus.) He appeared and he drank the hālāhala—he drank the poison that was generated by the initial process of inquiring into the truth; however, he did not swallow the poison. Instead he suspended the toxin in his throat, neither swallowing nor spitting it out. Not accepting or rejecting the initial poison that surfaced as a result of inquiry into the truth,

Śiva simply let the hālāhala rest right at his throat, and according to the myth, one of the foundational paradoxes of yoga was established —the poison was consumed but not swallowed. This act of simply letting the poison be within the bright, attentive, radiant space of the throat transmuted the poison into insight. In the process it caused Śiva's throat to turn blue, which is why one of the names of Śiva is Nīla Kaṇṭha, or the blue-throated one. Through contemplation on the two lotus feet of the guru—by allowing seemingly contrary perspectives to arise without swallowing them and without spitting them out—we find that the hālāhala of saṁsāra, the poison of conditioned existence, dissipates. In this way the two lotus feet of the guru provide shelter from the pangs of emotion associated with the complexity of existence and the fear of impermanence. It is these very same metaphorical feet that awaken the innate happiness of pure being, which is simply accepting the condition of things just as they are.

Perhaps one of the most accessible references to the guru, among many within yogic teachings, is that appearing in the *Bhāvana Upaniṣad* in which the guru is described as the suṣumnā nāḍī, or the central channel of the yogic body. The suṣumnā nāḍī, which begins in deep in the basin of the pelvis, just above the center of the pelvic floor, corresponds to the plumb line within your own body, of which you may become aware when you are standing or sitting straight. It rises, piercing through different planes of the body, up through the core of the heart, and on out through the crown of the head. It is hollow like a reed and is said to be empty, with no identifiable form at its core. This, of course, is just an approximate explanation of what is meant by the suṣumnā nāḍī, because it is from the core of the suṣumnā that all is thought to be generated, so words cannot accurately describe it. Somewhat like the heart of the sun, the suṣumnā nāḍī is looked upon as being empty, yet so full that it continuously generates endless experience and an infinity of worlds. Within all types of traditional yoga, the practices are designed to allow us to open up this central channel of the body and to cultivate a visceral connection within ourselves to a sense of truth from which all else flows. Through these practices we slowly start to realize that the suṣumnā nāḍī possesses a tremendous gravity and beauty that draw us in, and in that way its nature is that of the guru. We are drawn in and we surrender into the central channel because of this irresistible attractive quality. You could describe it as if we fall head over heels into the unknown, into the arms of the beloved, who is inside the central channel and the core of the heart. Once our internal breath, the prāṇa, enters the central channel, time and space are eaten by the immensity of this gravity. We find that the external guru, the person we have identified as our teacher (who could be an actual traditional guru—someone who is accomplished in the formal yogic arts—or who could simply be a clear-minded teacher), has always merely been pushing us toward our own central channel with the hopes that eventually we will fall right into it. Therefore a good teacher will use various tricks, techniques, or theoretical teachings in order to free you from the very things that keep you stuck in a belief system based on needing to know everything. A good teacher turns your attention toward the truth so that you no longer find comfort in, nor can you hide in, an avoidance of the unknown and in a surface presentation of the present moment. The guru points in whatever direction is necessary to direct you to exactly what it is that will allow you to be wide awake with raw, pure attention to whatever might occur in the immediate experience of "now." It is said that there are an unlimited number of gurus, or you could say that the one guru is saying the same thing in an unlimited number of languages and from an endless number of perspectives. The message of all of those perspectives is that the true self or the true nature of existence lies at the core of all beings and is beyond thought and language. It is beyond the forms that are generated and it is not different than those forms. Being beyond language, it is, paradoxically, the root subject of language. You cannot talk about it; however, it is the only thing that is really worth talking about.

A question that burns in the minds and hearts of many students is what happens if you do not have a good guru, and in fact, how do you know for sure whether a guru is actually first-rate? Various tools, in particular intuition, can be helpful in this light. If someone claims to be a guru (which in and of itself should be a warning signal), you should be particularly rigorous in your assessment as to whether the teacher exhibits clear thinking in their actions toward and in their relationships with others, as well as whether they seem to possess a depth of knowledge and understanding of the classical teaching as well as the practical applications of yoga. You should also practice careful self-reflection to discover whether the teacher is in some way hooking into your own ego as a means of building their image in your eyes through your adoration and surrender to them. This is the relationship teachers sometimes impose on their students, and it is a sign of an immature and nonskilled teacher. Good teachers are not detached from the world nor do they appear to be above others; instead, true gurus have a deeply rooted and vast sense of compassion and insight, and they function in the world with openness and respect for others. These are things that are sometimes difficult to read correctly—especially if a teacher is wanting (consciously or not) to attract followers. Part of the tradition of a guru-student relationship is that the questioning mind is encouraged and welcomed. That way, not only is the student examining the depths of the subject, but the relationship itself becomes the litmus test for whether or not the teachings and the guru are being approached and maintained as part of a bigger context of insight. The student must be encouraged to actually think about the subject matter, read original texts, and contemplate their meaning, and most important, the student must be guided in practicing the tradition as a means of actually experiencing firsthand the essence of the teachings. The teacher is responsible for honestly communicating with the student, and part of that honesty is that the guru continues studying and practicing as well. In addition, the teacher must guide the student correctly toward the root of the teaching rather than blinding the student to the essence of the teaching as a method of self-aggrandizement for the guru. This is at the root of all good teaching and is critical within the yogic tradition that rests so thoroughly in relationship.

Within the tradition of yoga, and as if triangulating, we rely on the plurality of others who are also practicing in order to gain a sense of direction for ourselves. It is said within the Hindu yogic tradition that we follow guru, the sādhu, and the śāstra. This is something like having three branches of government—the executive, legislative, and the judicial branches—and it allows for a system of checks and balances. The guru is the primary teacher and also brings knowledge and focus of the particular methodology or the lineage of teachings as you apply them to your unique circumstances. Sādhu simply means "holy person" and refers to the wide variety of people who are also within a lineage, or within distinct lineages or even separate religious disciplines. There is a remarkable similarity between people who have very distinct practices (or religions), but who also have deep insight into the core of the heart—a connection to the nature of reality. The similarity is recognizable in the type of smile you see on their faces and the quality of alertness reflected in their eyes; they are open, clear, content, compassionate, and deeply connected to all that is happening before their eyes. Resting in the often unspoken support of others who themselves are also in search of the truth is an important element in sustaining a deep and evolving inquiry into yoga. The third branch is the śāstra, which means the scriptures. Of course each lineage of yoga has its unique sets of scriptures, but there are also large bodies of scriptures that are accepted by nearly all lineages (both Hindu and Buddhist). So for students who have a good teacher and the inspiration from others on the path, it is also imperative to continue to study directly from the original texts—to read and contemplate the philosophical questioning and theorizing that has evolved over thousands of years. Within the Buddhist tradition there is also a threefold system that supports practitioners, that is, the Buddha, who could be considered to be the archetype of the guru; the saṅgha, which is the community of other practitioners and is equivalent to the sādhu; and the dharma, which means the teachings and practice, represented in the actual texts or śāstra of the Buddhist tradition.

With three reference points for finding a suitable guru and methodology, you are more likely to stay grounded within the core of your exploration into the meaning of life and into your own practice. It is not always easy to find this triangulation of support. Especially in the modern world we may have little access to a sādhu or even to other experienced practitioners of yoga. Unless we speak Sanskrit, or have found good translations of the traditional teachings, it may be equally difficult to access the original teachings of the śāstra. Finding a guru can be the most difficult task because many contemporary teachers are new to the subject and have not weathered the test of time. Some others may have had a mystical experience through yoga, they may have had deep insight into the meaning of reality, but have not taken off the training wheels of their particular sect. We may also find a teacher who is not deeply accomplished in the yogic arts but who is taking advantage of the great desire many people have to learn yoga. The teacher may play off of the egos of students, manipulating them in ways that are unethical and unkind. This is a particularly sad situation within the context of yoga because many students come to this practice when they are in a vulnerable position in their lives and need to explore the subtleties of their own mind that are arising through the practices. These kinds of unethical teachers will systematically work so that you have no access to the original texts, to other lineages, or to other practitioners who might bring you back down to earth. Such teachers do not encourage students to question the ideas of the teaching or the actions and ideas that they present, instead telling students what to believe and often how to behave. Such behavior is a sign of an immature or unskilled teacher who does this sort of thing to boost their own ego. It is an age-old problem within any system that young, inexperienced teachers (or scoundrels masquerading as teachers) manipulate students and the teachings themselves in these ways. So beware and trust your instincts when looking for a guru and a lineage.

Remember that yoga is something that is real; as a tradition it is a continual synthesis of the experience of millions of practitioners—all of whom are essentially within the same boat of being surrounded by sensation, feeling, thought, and intelligence. All yoga traditions follow remarkably similar principles, no matter what particular language or specific culture lies at their root. Although it may be difficult to find a good teacher, the good news is that whether you do not have a good guru, or if you *do* have a good guru but are unaware of it, whether you love your guru even if your guru is not good, or if you do not love your guru in spite of the fact that your guru is actually very good—under any of these circumstances, all hope is not lost. The *principle* of relationship, the dual points of view that are merging into one perspective, reflected by the two feet of a multiplicity of gurus as well as in your relationship with your guru—*this* is what is important. The principle of relationship with the teacher is exactly parallel to the principle of relationship with anyone else; whether it is your girlfriend or boyfriend, your spouse, your parents, your children, your pets, or even random people on the street. Regardless of the specifics, the principle of relationship in which the interpenetrating nature of all phenomena is revealed remains the same.

We love to place our teacher or our guru on a pedestal. Just like our lovers, whom we also tend to place on a pedestal. That way they become the symbol in our heart for everything that we want: they embody our desire for freedom, beauty, and even for life itself. We think of them as we would beautiful music, blue skies, chirping birds, flowers, and springtime. This is a universal phenomenon. But be it our teacher or our lover, if we have placed them on the pedestal, we are engaged in reducing them to the theories we have about them. In so doing we want them to be exactly like the images of them that we hold hidden in our deepest mind. This does not allow us to truly experience the immense gravity of who they actually are or the boundless depth in the core of their hearts—that part to which we are instinctively attracted and the part that is inconceivable and inexpressible. When we place the teacher on a pedestal, we are conversely placing ourselves in a pit. It is as if the pedestal were created by digging space for it in the ground, leaving a depression, and we then go and stand in this hollow. In this way all of our innate intelligence—our questioning mind, clear vision, cleverness, and our skepticism—are given away. Through this process we become unintelligent and dependent on the image of what we now believe to be the teacher rather than inspired by the reality of the teachings. Under these circumstances we are not really in relationship with the guru, now on the pedestal, because we do not have an immediate awareness of their being or an immediate connection to and appreciation for the delicacy of life. We have fallen out of relationship with the person we call our teacher, and it is almost impossible under these circumstances for that person to be in a true relationship with us as well. The very practices of yoga have evolved through this incalculable synthesis of the working through of a relationship—with so many teachers and with so many students. This very amalgamation allows us to continue on even in the face of the natural process of transference of our own intelligence onto our teacher. It is the teacher's foremost duty to give you back your intelligence, to return to you your heart, to encourage you to access yourself. They do this by being who they really are, and by being completely honest and compassionate with you. It is in such an environment of absolute truth and trust that we find the actual process of yoga, one in which both teacher and student are honest about what they know and are sincerely willing to look at the processes of *how* they know what they know. Students will pick up this process from their teacher and then they will actually begin delving into the yoga, finding the truth and the guru deep in the core of their own hearts, just as their teacher has found her own guru within the core of her heart.

The process of yoga can be almost embarrassing when we become aware of our ignorance and the fact that we have made a projection. For example, even though we might have comprehended the concept of a guru as someone who through their teaching and actions points us to the truth found within in the present moment and within our own hearts, we might suddenly become aware of the fact that we have taken a form—someone, something, some technique—and that we have become idolaters by placing that form upon a pedestal. We might find that we have done this even within the context of the yoga practice itself! The embarrassing part is that in doing this we have actually stopped the real unfolding of yoga in order to create the appearance of the yogic process. When we hear about the phenomenon of the guru who becomes self-absorbed and manipulates his students, we probably think that we would never fall for such a transparent trick. But we may have unwittingly fallen for it in many subtle and insidious ways, because a universal phenomenon for all human beings is that we tend to give away our power to others. It is quite common to transfer onto a teacher, a parent, or a peer some aspect of our inquiry—this is the classic definition of transference or giving away our power to others. When we do this, in order to preserve the constructed mask of a relationship, in the process we wind up aborting our inquiry into what is real and true. Under these circumstances, supporting the illusion of the projections of our mind—the transference—feels almost like self-preservation. So we stop thinking deeply, looking at the truth, and inquiring into the nature of reality. As humans we love to jump to conclusions, to try to seal down reality, whether it is the reality of our own being or our idea of the reality of the totality of the universe.

The process of yoga and of relating to a guru leads to the discovery of the workings of our own mind. Perhaps the most common aspect of mind that is revealed through yoga is that of ignorance when it is defined as superimposing that which is limited, context dependent, and temporary onto that which is unlimited, infinite, and pure. Through this form of ignorance we project essence outward, and we become attached to outward form. For example, we see the guru as infallible and as being beyond human, or we have a mystical experience and believe that one experience separates us (and elevates us) from other "mortals," or we imagine that the form and structure of the practices we do are the essence of the teaching. The process of yoga is the practice of bringing conscious awareness to this very natural and reductive function of mind. You could say yoga is the drawing of a circle and then the erasing of that circle, which leads to drawing another circle that is again erased. Yoga is the ongoing process of creating a sacred space, then dissolving the borders of that sacred space, and then defining the sacred space again in the context of the most current and relevant moment in time. Ignorance, or avidyā, arises when we forget to erase the circle that we ourselves have created within our own mind, when we think our insight into the present moment is a permanent state of affairs. This is an incredibly powerful aspect of mind—that we can take an ordinary table and through the power of mind we can say, and fervently believe, that everything on that table is sacred. People do this symbolically all the time, for example, when they set up an altar and then become trapped by the power they have projected into the objects they place on the altar. This ability is certainly not all bad; it allows us to focus the mind as we reduce the vast complexity of existence to symbols or to simple metaphors that are understandable and are then easy to work with. In fact, this is what thinking is. A thought is an idea or a universal that allows us to place a large number of particular events into a box. For example, the idea "chair" is a universal concept, but there are actually thousands and potentially an unlimited number of particular, unique chairs. We can understand each chair as separate, and at the same time we can appreciate them all through a universal or an idea we name "chair." This organizational and thinking skill is basically what the mind is designed to do, but problems arise when we take its work of creating categories and concepts lierally. Once we have created a sacred space, and have empowered that space by defining what is inside the circle as sacred and what is outside the circle as irrelevant, then we make the mistake of taking our arbitrary definition literally. It is essential in the process of creating a sacred space (or any concept) to realize where that sacred space or the concept came from, and to then be able to consciously erase the borders of our definition. It is equally important to then create new borders when and if appropriate. This is the essence of the yogic process, and it is also the essence of how to have a real relationship with anyone else. In all that we do it is vitally important to look clearly again and again so that at the appropriate moment we are able to let go of our sacred circles, so that we can reevaluate our means of identifying situations and release our expectations. By letting go you can understand your concept's dependency on the context that you have defined within the system of your own mind, and in so doing you might possibly see things clearly as they are arising.

We develop this skill of defining and letting go through all aspects and phases of a balanced yoga practice. It is part of our training to be comfortable with not-knowing so that at the time of death, the sacred space that we have defined as our body can be allowed to dissolve. If the yogic process is fully awakened, then death is actually considered to be an excellent event—a joyous time. But if we identify with the forms we have created within our minds, if we cling to our ideas of sacred space, then great fear arises at the moment of dissolution. In other words, if someone who is dying identifies the "self" as the immediate physical and mental experiences occurring at the time of death, if a person identifies the physical body as the "self," then there is great fear at the prospect of dissolution. The fear of dissolution of the self and of the ego may be greatest at the time of death, but it arises in less extreme circumstances all the time. When the yoga practice starts to really work and our image of ourselves as totally separate from everything else begins to dissolve, we become deeply aware of others. This can be a good thing as it can lead to insight, compassion, and the ability to live with not-knowing. But whenever we meet something that lies outside of our system (and our system would be defined as our body, mind, feelings, sensations, thoughts, emotions) there is also the potential for conflict and a very real possibility of resistance to the dissolution of our defined system "self," which can result in feelings of great fear. Our system is the ego, the part of ourselves we believe to be separate and permanent, and it is also the part of ourselves that allows us to feel secure and certain in the world. So when we meet something outside of our own defined system—for example, another person who happens to have a prominent ego, someone involved in another religion, or someone from another culture—in order to interact with the "other" and to have an authentic relationship with them, we *must* dissolve at least some of the boundaries of our own "system." We must soften the boundaries of our ego enough to allow holes in the borders of our sacred spaces and those things we have identified ourselves with, so that we can actually interface in some way with the other. The paradox is that it is equally important, after dissolving our borders in a relationship, to redefine them and then to redissolve them again and again and again.

So it is with our relationship to the teacher, the guru: someone who initially appears to us as the other. Once we have incorporated them into our own system—merged the corner of their ideas with our own, considered that their perspective is at least as authentic as our own, once we have shared some laughter together—then we think we know who they are, and we may even begin to identify with them, and it is at this moment that we must redefine the borders of our own self. It is the guru's duty at that juncture in the relationship to drop back and to appear as the other, the unknown, thereby reestablishing the boundaries in order that they again may be dissolved. We continuously have to dissolve and reconnect, then restructure and disperse again, our sacred spaces, those things that we tend to identify with.

When two things meet, it is right there at their conjunction that yoga occurs. It is said that when day meets night, when in-breath meets out-breath, *this* is where yoga appears. This is because it is in that initial communication, in that process of two systems meeting, that each system has to dissolve. Each system must release its identification with itself; it must let go of the baggage it carries, reconsider its techniques, release all of its temporary concepts and all of the limited aspects that it has identified as its own separate essence. Whether it is a person, a religion, or a corporation, any system must drop back into its true nature in order to experience the other. Through connection with the other—through yoga—we find our true selves. This is why the yoga tradition has been passed on from teacher to student and from student to teacher. It is passed on through a healthy relationship with the other, and it flourishes through finding the essence of that teacher-student relationship that reveals the essence of all relationships. It is not absolutely essential that the yoga teacher be perfect, meaning that they conform to a particular set of standards. Better that the yoga teacher is able to create and dissolve sacred spaces, that she has opened her heart and has understood that the real bottom line lies in the union of ideas, in the joining of opposites, and in authentic relationships with the others. A good teacher is able to continuously restart his own practice of yoga and to drop back to the very beginning. Through a good teacher's presence others are able to relax and to drop back as well. A good teacher simply allows us to be comfortable enough that we are able to observe the process of our own mind, which is this process of making idols, of making mistakes, superimpositions, and transferences. In seeing this process and in observing it in the light of the necessity of true relationship, by allowing ourselves to gradually and continuously let it go, then day by day—perhaps even moment by moment—we can awaken to the present moment.

If you are a teacher, this means that you have to have a teacher, and that teacher in turn has to have a teacher. The chain of teachers is to be imagined as going back endlessly, which allows the teacher of the teachers—or the present moment—to be the true source of the teaching. These lineages of teachers are often imagined as the guru sitting inside of the crown of the head of the student. The image continues so that inside of that teacher's head, sits another guru, and so it goes back into an endless chain of teachers and endless linking of relationship. If you are a teacher, you must practice surrender. As a teacher, more than anyone, you are willing to give up your preconceptions about what is and to simply be in awe of a process that you do not truly understand but that you intuit as the very heart of your own existence. So to be a teacher, humility is the requirement, and entering into the suṣumnā nāḍī is the process of finding that humility. In this way you automatically respect students, and you are able to give students back to themselves continuously, even if they insist on projecting or transferring aspects of themselves and their beliefs onto you. You give it all back to them automatically. As a teacher, at no point do you actually identify with the role of "teacher" because in that identification there is an enormous risk of ego inflation. So the good news for most, and the bad news for a few, is that being a yoga teacher, a guru, is not a career path. The guru is an archetype, and there is no need for the ego to identify and to become possessed by that archetype.

If you are a student, having a teacher means that you have realized that the process of life and the process of yoga are beyond your ability to completely control. Even though you may intuitively know you are so close to understanding life, deep inside your heart you also know that the true mystery of life and of the present moment is revealed only through surrender, through letting go, through not controlling and not-knowing. To be able to simply rest and to fall back into the very nature of existence, to be able to dissolve into the core of pure being without having to hold on to any belief or any conceptual system or form, to release any hope and attachment to finding reality, *this* is the essential practice of yoga. To become a student is to become a fool, and to become a fool is to become wise.

In this light, truly nothing we can come up with, no matter how bizarre, lies outside of the realm of yoga practice. Yoga is the release of all things through the cultivation of insight into the heart of all things. It is said that perfection in yoga can come very quickly, perhaps immediately to someone who surrenders to the guru—which is exactly what Kṛṣṇa told Arjuna in the Bhagavad Gītā. A yogi is one who trusts in the truth of pure love, one who drops into all experience as it arises, trusting the essence of the heart, which enables the yogi to offer all experience, particularly the core experience of the mind, into the fire of awareness. It is this fire of awareness that is the true guru. This form of surrender means an ability to see that even our innermost thoughts and feelings are part of a completely natural and shared process. It is said that everything, particularly *this* (meaning what you are experiencing right now), whether it is the feeling in your knees or in your hand, or the particular thoughts in your head, all of *this* is enveloped by the principle of the guru—the principle of the guru of gurus. When you realize that whatever you are experiencing—*this*—is not yours, there is a great sense of relief, and you can let it go. You can observe it without accepting it or rejecting it, just as Śiva was able to take in the hālāhala, the poison of existence, without swallowing it and without spitting it back out. In this letting go as if it was not yours, you find incredible happiness with an astonishing pleasure of pure being; you find the natural radiant joy that is yoga.

Sometimes after hearing about the different types of yoga practice, after listening to the teachings of the Upaniṣads and contemplating how deep the truth of our own existence must be, we feel at a loss as to how to actually begin the practice of yoga. This is a natural response. But again, taking a step backward, releasing our grip of identity with ourselves and with our own very real experiences, can be a huge relief. One of the most important aspects of viewing yoga as being a matrix of interpenetrating ideas, thoughts, and experiences is that it provides the image of an interwoven safety net that lies beneath us, and each joining of the net reflects our own experience of the process of yoga itself. It provides the support of knowing that everything is connected, which makes the prospect of stepping back and letting go, while also welcoming an opportunity to start over, interesting rather than daunting. The view of yoga as a matrix allows us to return to the very beginning of the practice again and again and again because we need not accumulate embellishments to our ego in the form of yoga practice.

There is really no hierarchy of achievement, ranking, or levels of attainment that we should take too seriously in the practice of yoga.

There is not that much that actually needs to be remembered on the spot, but there *is* something much more essential within our hearts that is inspired through yoga; it is always present and available wherever we are. Within the course of our yoga practice we often find we've come to a point where our study has left us dry, as if washed up on a beach. We may get to this stage when we sense how far-reaching and deep the truth is; it may seem as though there is an impossible gap between where we find ourselves and where we imagine it all leading. We may feel as if there is no technique, no mantra, no desire, nothing that could possibly bridge that endless gap between ourselves and the truth. In coming to this point we are offered the important opportunity to start over with the practice, to find out what our original motivation for practicing yoga was, and then to look at what is actually happening. Junctures such as these are an open invitation to go back to the breath, and through the breath to go back to the sensations that are occurring in our body. By steadying the mind in those sensations, we can then observe the pattern of our thoughts, the very pattern that our ego is composed of, and once again we find ourselves entering the web that is the practice of yoga.

A common confusion for yoga students is to wonder what type of practice is best. Should I practice bhakti yoga since I am a person of very strong emotions? Should I practice jñāna yoga since I love to think about things, I love to understand things? Should I practice the postures of haṭha yoga because the posture and breathing practices are very tangible? Should I practice tantra yoga because I am a person of great desire and of insatiable lust—perhaps I can dovetail those energies into finding the truth of my own existence? We have seen through this brief exploration of the yoga tradition that all teachings point out that every type of practice is actually a composite of other types of practice. However you wish to label yourself, whatever school you align with, if you go deeply into any form you will eventually find that you are doing all of the different types of yoga through the form you have chosen. This is probably the most important teaching of the *Bhagavad Gītā* for those who have become deeply enmeshed in yoga practices. You can call yourself a bhakta or a devotee one day, and the next day call yourself a jñāni, or one who practices the art of wisdom. Likewise, when practicing yoga poses, calling yourself a haṭha yogi you may wonder what pose you should be doing next, but as you continue through the āsanas you may begin to see that as you practice any of the poses and remain sensitive to your circumstances, you naturally begin to adjust the body on a deep internal level. You begin to see that it is not so much specifically which pose you do or how deeply you get into any one of the poses that is of greatest import, rather that your awareness of breath and your ability to truly connect to the inner feelings and sensations that draw you back into the heart of the practice are what matter. When you approach a yoga practice with an open mind and a true passion for being present with and meeting whatever arises, you know that if you go deeply into any of the different disciplines, you are going to bring all of the other disciplines in as well.

Practicing yoga is not always easy. Sometimes the biggest difficulty is arranging a time to do it: starting the session of practice. But if you can trick yourself into just beginning, it often works out. If you have arranged a time to practice but do not really feel like practicing, the trick is to convince yourself to simply stand up in samasthitiḥ, to take three breaths, thinking that you will allow yourself to go off and do something else after that simple ritual. Then after standing in samasthitiḥ, it often turns out that the idea of taking a big inhale, raising your arms and doing half of a sun salutation is alluring. Having done that, one full sun salutation before quitting may seem reasonable. Soon you may find yourself doing two, and then three sun salutations; and then all of a sudden, you are in the groove and the practice continues. One reason the practice can be difficult is that the mind is a very strict taskmaster, and it often creates images of what practice is or it should be. The parameters your own mind sets for the practice may erode the foundation of the practice itself; if you cannot do a "good" practice, why practice at all? You may think to yourself that if you are going to sit in meditation, you must sit for forty-five minutes. If you are going to practice prāṇāyāma, you should practice it for one hour, and that if you are going to practice āsana, two hours is the minimum. When, in fact, if you were to do any of these practices with true concentration even for two seconds, you would open up the core of the body and have remarkable insight and a sense of freedom—particularly a sense of release from the game you have constructed in your mind of what practicing is. Again, we run into the notion of drawing a circle (defining the parameters of our practice) and erasing the circle (having mercy on ourselves if we cannot meet the standards we have set for ourselves). For beginning students, allowing some leeway in some of the parameters we set for ourselves about the structure and consistency of our practice can be the golden ticket to jump-start a routine of practice that, once it is going, automatically draws you back day after day, year after year. Of course, for longtime practitioners, those of us whose minds have comprehended the "draw a circle and erase it" metaphor, the trick may be to encourage ourselves to stick with the parameters we or our teacher have suggested a little longer before erasing the circle, before sabotaging our practice by skipping the parts we do not like. There is a time for perseverance, and there is a time to release the reins of the mind: a time to stick precisely with the parameters, and a time to recognize the effect of the circumstances of our own life on the boundaries that are established. It is all called being mindful of what is actually arising rather than being attached to what we think is or what we want to be arising.

If we look at each type of practice as a well to be dug, as we dig deeper and deeper we start to find that the other practices are involved in making the hole truly deep. So we may start out with the practice of haṭha yoga, committing ourselves to the opening up of the body, the stretching out of the prāṇa, and the uniting of prāṇa and the apāna in order to open the central channel so that our breath will flow smoothly and freely. As we go deeper into the haṭha yoga practice we become more sensitive, and soon we find that we are actually practicing tantra. Tantric practice brings us into proximity or identification with our beloved deity, and we find ourselves concerned with bhakti and indifferent to kuṇḍalinī and mantra. Bhakti yoga shows us that the various āsanas, the various prāṇāyāmas, have everything to do with our relationships to our teacher, to other people, and how we interact with the world around us. As we go deeper into relating to others we find that actually we are practicing jñāna yoga, because in our relationships we must look deeply into who others truly are. In order to maintain this understanding of the true nature of others, we realize that we must loosen the grip we have on our ideas about them, so that our preconceptions and desires do not interfere with our relationships. Going deeper still into jñāna yoga, we again find ourselves back practicing haṭha yoga. As we think, so we feel; as we think, so we posture the body; and by re-posturing, re-visioning the positioning of the body and the breath, we find that we refresh the mind, and we are able to uncover the emotional and habitual roots of our thinking patterns. So the cycle goes on and on, and not only do we end up practicing all the different types of yoga, but we practice all the different limbs of aṣṭāṅga yoga and various combinations and sequences of practice within those types and those limbs.

When we choose to begin the practice of yoga by fixing our attention on whatever form of yoga we are practicing, as we go deeper into the actual practice we start to discover that everything rests within a nest and is dependent on its context. Initially we learn to focus our mind. Whether we focus on the action of our kneecap in a yoga pose, or on the dominance of breath in one of our nostrils, or whether we focus our mind on a pattern of our emotions or of our thoughts, after the mind is focused a kind of tension arises. This tension is what we know as tapas or heat. Even in everyday life, you can periodically feel heat building internally when you really focus on what you are doing. Through practicing we notice that if we maintain the tapas without a strong sense of repulsion or desire, the context of whatever we have chosen to meditate on is revealed. Essentially, we begin to sense that whatever has become the focus of our awareness is interpenetrating, through a unified background, into everything else we might think, feel, or perceive. This is a fundamental principle of a yoga practice: that when we focus the mind—no matter what the content of that focus—eventually the very content that we have chosen as the focus begins to reveal its background. This is easy to understand if we imagine what it is like when we focus on the tip of an iceberg; very soon we intuit that it is simply the tip of something that is much deeper. The iceberg as the object of our attention interpenetrates everything else. In the same way, if we choose a point of intersection in a net, we discover at that very point there exist connections to the entire net. In the mythical Jeweled Net of Indra, at each point of intersection in the net, there is a jewel that reflects all of the other jewels, all of the other points of intersection. This myth offers a beautiful image of the way the world actually works, of the interpenetration of all aspects of life. With practice we begin to see that what appears to be separate—that which is our present experience—is not actually detached and separate at all. When we pay close attention in a meditative manner to whatever our present experience is, all of a sudden we sense its interdependence with everything else. By allowing the mind to settle into the present moment we are able to see that our "separate" experience is really resting in this vast net we call life. In this way, the practice of yoga always reveals context, and when context is revealed there is an incredible sense of release and relaxation. It is as if things are being taken care of. We can see that the responsibility for the maintenance of the body, the mind, in fact the maintenance of the entire world, is no longer resting on the shoulders of the flimsy ego. All is actually taken care of by this vast substratum, and the nature of this bedrock is something that yoga theory has contemplated for centuries.

By continually reformulating our theories about what the actual medium we are working with is, some schools of Indian philosophy have the point of resting in the understanding that the matrix is actually Brahman or pure consciousness. Brahman simply has the qualities of sat, which means "truth" or "permanence," cit, which is "consciousness," and ānanda, or "joy." So we could say, metaphorically, that the universe is like a tapestry composed of many thousands of threads that intersect in an infinite number of places, and that if we look at any one of those threads, we find that the very center of that thread is hollow like a tube. We discover that the nature of that empty thread, in fact the very nature of the space within that thread—that which allows life to flow—is relationship. So it turns out that relationship is the one aspect of yoga that keeps the practice grounded. You could become very skilled at yoga postures, at philosophy, or at prāṇāyāma, but still, when it comes to relating to someone else, you could be a beginner. This is true for everyone. We are, all of us, *always* beginners in relationship because to relate to another, someone outside the systems of our own mind and our own ego, we must temporarily suspend those very systems that we so closely identify with, and we must come back to the beginning. We must release our theories in order to connect in the present moment with someone else.

It is important to recognize that through connection with others we naturally upgrade and return to our own systems of knowledge; we do and should continue to use the structures of our ego in order to relate to others, but we must also be able to let them go. If we are dominated by our structures, then we are unable to interact outside of our own ego and we cannot dissolve into the web of support that is yoga, so that ultimately we experience a sense of separation, fear, and suffering. Most often, what we are afraid of is the truth. We are fearful of the clear vision revealed through yoga that the body and mind are simply vibration. It can be confusing if not frightening to contemplate the notion that all things that we can identify as being ourselves and everything we see as distinctly ours are actually not separate at all. There is no "us," but instead all of it is an interpenetrating aspect of every*one* and every*thing* else. When we grasp the vision of being identifiable individuals who are also literally part of everything else, then we can actually see, just as Arjuna was able to see through the story of the *Bhagavad Gītā*, that the universe is a kind of death machine in which everything is impermanent. Initially this vision is terrifying, and it marks the very beginning of deep yoga practice, when there is a visceral understanding of the truth that we are all in the same basic situation with our bodies and minds. Moment by moment we are facing death, that of our own body along with the death and the transformation of everybody and everything that we know. This underlying teaching of the *Bhagavad Gītā* is the initial key teaching of yoga as relationship.

It is said that someone is a real practitioner of yoga when she is able to see the true self, the ātman, in everyone, while at the same time seeing all others in the ātman. The essence of our vision of yoga, therefore, is that in a very deep and radical sense, we are all the same being. This yogic insight, however, exists within a layer of our awareness that often remains mysterious because it is a level beyond the formulations of the mind, outside the realm of that which is perceivable. The extent of our interrelatedness with others and all aspects of the world can be a truly alarming vision. We see that the body we consider to be ourselves is actually a tiny speck, intermeshed with this very delicate biological web that is temporarily covering the surface of the planet Earth, and if you look closely you may see that it is a very unstable and temporary situation. We begin to see that even our very own multifaceted insights and our profound desires are simply part of a cultural net, a shared latticework that is not really unique to our own particular ego. It turns out that the conditioned mind's worst perceptions of reality provide the impetus to actually wake up. When we discover that we are really each other and that our own dearly beloved body is enmeshed in the very fabric of the universe, then there is a release of the mind's multi-pointed focusses and the arising of clear, one-pointed focus, defined in the *Yoga Sūtra* as samādhi pariṇāma, or transformation samādhi. It begins the uncovering of the actual nature of the matrix as being an absolute freedom, a radiant, limitless ecstasy, described as both complete aloneness and a sense of being enmeshed. So, we are completely separate from and intimately connected to everything else, both at the same time. As we have seen, in the *Yoga Sūtra*, suffering is said to be grounded in avidyā or in the ignorance of pure consciousness, being mistaken for that which is impermanent and with a limited form. It is an ignorance grounded in identification with false self. The last root of suffering, abhiniveśa, is when through ignorance we cling irrationally and spontaneously to life. Abhiniveśa is said to arise even in the minds of those who are very wise. If we can allow the wave of fear at the thought of being not separate from all else to wash through us, we then find that the very vibration of this insight is the clear light of reality. That which was the most terrifying aspect of reality turns out to give us the greatest joy. The thing we choose to rarely talk or think about, but which is really the only guaranteed thing in life—the fact that we will die—can truly draw us into the present moment. It splits open our hearts and gives us true relationship because it reveals the mysterious and deep nature of relationship as a sustaining aspect of reality.

If we go through a lifetime of yoga practice, if we memorize the Upaniṣads and can do every conceivable yoga posture, if we are able to hold our breath for three hours, and we acquire all kinds of titles as a yoga master, even if we become famous throughout the three worlds for our practice of yoga—where is all of this at the end of our life? At the time of death, when you are choking on mucous, where is your prāṇāyāma? When the central nervous system is failing, how important is it that you stretch those hamstring muscles you have been working on for years? When we are facing death, these things reveal their true nature: that they are enmeshed in an interwoven matrix of all else that is life in the infinite reaches of the universe. Whether it is at the moment of death, or right now, *this* is our chance; it is the moment when we can begin the practice of yoga again. The opportunity to start over at the very beginning is always available, but we often overlook it. We may build the edifices of the ego in the mind for years and years and years before we see through them, before we actually use those very structures of mind as the object of our meditation. But then, through practice, context is revealed. By practicing, by starting over, the context of whatever the focus of the practice is becomes revealed more frequently. This is a gradual process; in the beginning, maybe once every five years we really face the games that we are playing. Then perhaps we meet our illusions of mind twice a year, then maybe twice a month we get back to a grounded reality, a real yoga practice. Eventually twice a week or three times a day we are able to let go of our mind games and get back to the present moment. Gradually the frequency increases until perhaps every five minutes; or if we are skilled, maybe every two or three seconds we start over, stepping out of our games of preconception and avoidance of the present moment. Again and again we look at reality with fresh, innocent eyes, open ears, and an open heart, until the process of waking up becomes like a hum in the background of all existence, *the* frequency that underlies everything. Eventually the letting go into the present circumstance metaphorically becomes like the hum of the syllable *oṁ,* and that very nature of the mind, releases the mind. This is the theme of tantra; it is the mind that releases the mind, it is the knowable that shows us the unknowable. The immediate things that are happening in your life—and many of the things that are happening are deeply rooted in confusion and suffering—these very same things are the medicine that is going to end your own suffering.

Once we have insight into this aspect of the nature of being and of mind, no matter how esoteric or advanced we become in our study of yoga, we find that it is the practice and the releasing of that same practice in a continuous cycle that remains the key to freedom. At a certain level of understanding we must see through what we are doing until we recognize that it is all simply the guṇas of prakṛti acting upon the guṇas of prakṛti. Understanding this does not mean that we have "got it" and that therefore we should abandon our practice (though that is often the instinct at this phase of the practice), because the practice is an expression of the matrix and is the very activity of life itself. At the same time, within a healthy yoga practice we do not become stuck in the particulars, nor do we become shackled by our theories about it. We release, deepen, and refine the practice so that we do not identify with it and do not use it for selfish ends. This is why it is very helpful to engage in service to others within the context of your yoga practice: because it places everything in perspective.

Even without a formal yoga practice all of us are already practicing, doing things all of the time, and this is one of the ironies of yoga; we are all doing yoga whether we want to or not. We are constantly creating little idols in our mind, serving the idols, and occasionally knocking them over to build new ones. Everyone who has a mind does this all the time. From this perspective, since we are already practicing, a formal yoga practice just slows down to reveal to us what is already happening. As we hone the skill of bringing awareness to the subtleties of the present moment, the puruṣa (pure consciousness) is awakening into clear observation of a process that is already happening. We then see that the interpenetration of all things within the field before us is the mother ground of practice, and we truly comprehend that at the core of all practice is this insight into the nature of relationship as being at the heart of every aspect of existence. This understanding inevitably brings practice back to earth and grounds it in simple honesty. So yoga is a very human activity. Advancement is not measured in terms of siddhis, or magical powers, or in fame or political powers. Instead advancement in yoga is measured as honesty, as insight into the very foundation of knowledge based in the core of the heart. It is also measured by vairāgyam, or

non attamment

nonattachment, the ability to let things go. Just as the sun lets its energy go all the time, so too the advanced yoga practitioner is constantly letting his philosophy and beliefs go while engaging in the practices with a feeling of continuous, radiant release. An advanced yoga practitioner does not have to appear to be untouchable and exotic, or extraordinarily unique. Instead someone deeply steeped in and accomplished at the practice becomes more accessible, more normal and ordinary, more human on all fronts.

So whenever we look at yoga practice, whether it is our own or the practice of another, we know that jñāna, or wisdom, and vairāgyam, nonattachment, are the fruits of true practice. We know that perhaps someone can walk on water, they might be immensely famous and popular, and maybe they can pontificate about esoteric philosophies that are incomprehensible, but none of these count for anything in terms of the world of true relationship, true yoga. Given this, we might wonder what is the importance of philosophy and why we should worry about studying it at all. The answer is that philosophy is not restricted to theories debated and recorded in ancient texts; it is an innate human activity that all of us are doing all of the time. We are always thinking. We are constantly making theories about the world, testing them out, and even revising them occasionally. All of us are philosophers even if the academic subject seems repulsive to us and even if we may not be accomplished. Philosophy is the essential catalyst for the practice of yoga since it is the function of mind. When we study philosophy we see that it is not really an opinion, or a theory, but rather that philosophy is concerned with the world as it is; it is the study of how things really are in the world. So when we practice any type of yoga we are actually practicing philosophy, and through this we learn to cultivate the skill of releasing the practice itself so that, whether we are doing a yoga pose or philosophizing about life itself, we learn to start over at ground zero again and again and again. The job of philosophy is to allow us to experience the body as it is, to see the mind in its natural state, to see others as they are, to see the world around us just as it is. Good philosophy encourages a full multiplicity of viewpoints, and it allows us to explore new perspectives so that we become free of philosophizing altogether.

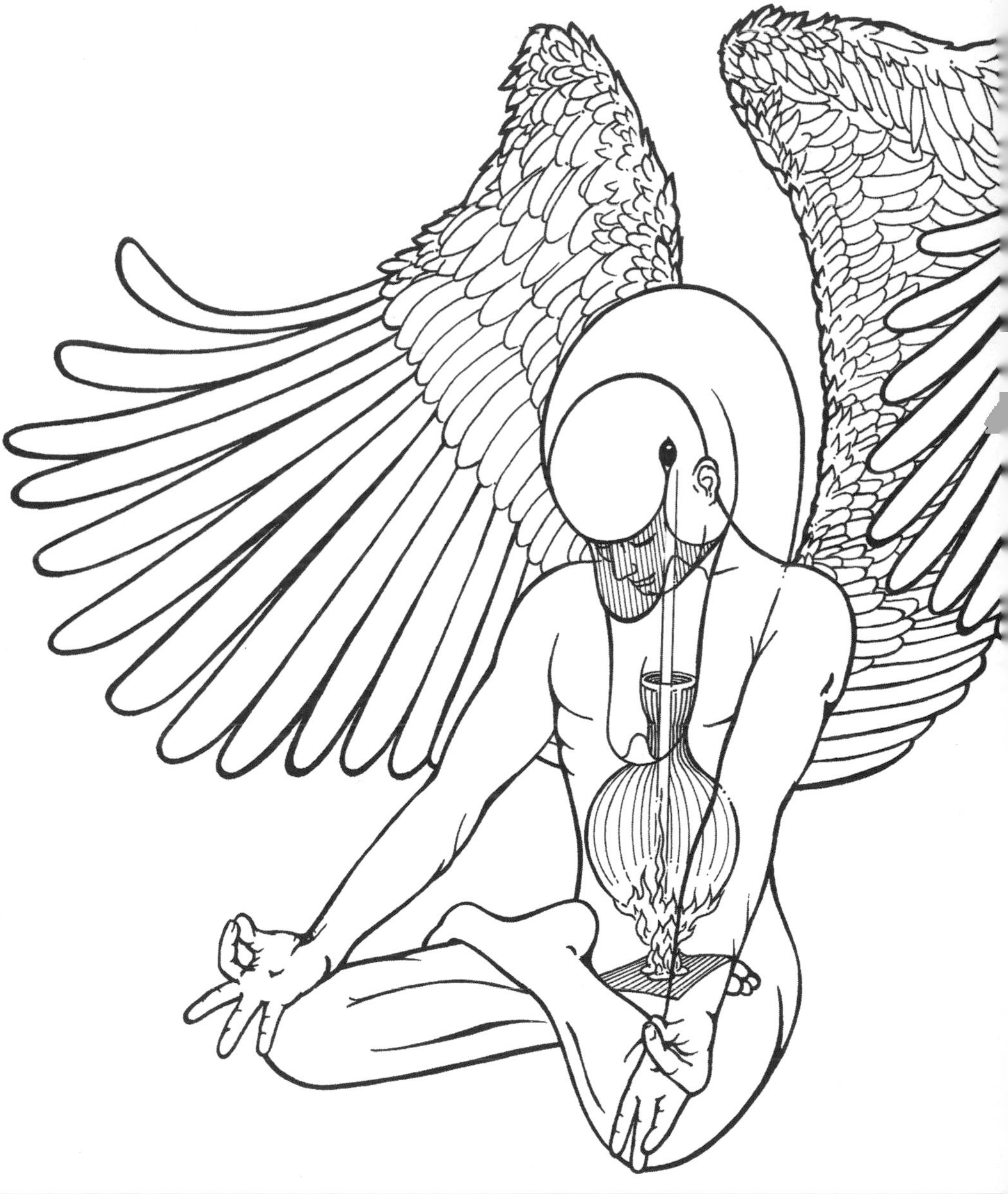

The word *philosophy* is actually a composite of two Greek words: *philo*, which means "love," and *sophia,* which means "wisdom," so you could imagine philosophy to be either the wisdom of love or the love of wisdom. Both views, when joined together, give us freedom. It is so easy to get carried away or lost in our ideas and our fantasies, but when we realize that yoga's jeweled net is actually the human body, our own human body, then our perspectives may still shift, but our mind can settle. By entering the jeweled net by means of that which is most immediate and real to us, all of our ideas, perceptions, feelings, and sensations can be brought home, giving us a direct and tangible experience of what yoga actually is. So when we talk about joining together wisdom and love, or linking the gem of the known with the matrix of the unknown, of connecting form with context—we can actually experience it in a down-to-earth, practical, real way. If we consider for a moment the joining together of apāna and prāṇa—the rooting and the flowering patterns, we see that they they are utterly interdependent. This uniting of the inhaling and the exhaling patterns allows us to feel the residue of each in the other, which reveals the suṣumnā nāḍī at the core of the body. Feeling this central axis we can access deep emotion, and we can experience our thoughts rooted in sensation, feeling, and deep memory. So truly, it is through these movements of prāṇa and apāna that the mind becomes embodied as *our* body. Likewise the habits of perception

Swan at the Pot of the Belly (8)

The swan represents the liberated ātman. It floats on the clear, calm lake of the enlightened mind. When the swan sleeps it rests its head on its heart in samādhi. The shape illustrated here is formed by the practice of mūlabandha, uḍḍiyāna bandha, and jālandhara bandha. These bandhas unite the prāṇa and the apāna which then interpenetrate and fully spread into this integrated shape, opening the back of the diaphragm like wings while opening the center of the heart like a buoyant sun. This integration and suspension of the in-breath and the out-breath ignites a fire under the pot of the belly, opens the vacuous, bright tube of the central channel, allowing the mind to rest in its own radiant nature, free of conceptual coverings.

in the body and the movements of the body are, in a very deep way, constantly influencing the fluctuations and patterns of our mind. This means that yoga can be practiced under all circumstances. It might not be the form of a yoga practice that your mind flatters itself into thinking it should be doing; you might be laid up in the hospital, or you might be like Arjuna and involved in an extremely complex political crisis, but you can still do yoga.

The very presence of your breath and of your body is one of the most astonishing things in the universe, and it offers the continual opportunity to start over. This awareness allows us to start the entire project of our life over, to reinitiate all the threads of our thought, grounding it all in the immediate experience of the body. What an incredible relief it is to understand that the ultimate place of pilgrimage is right in the center of our very own heart. The realization of the simple fact of the existence of our own body can be a source of the greatest joy, even though we know that the body as we know it is subject to birth, disease, old age, and death. In spite of the fact that the body is enmeshed in a network of biological dependency, of craving, hatred, and ego, encapsulated in a very false concept of ourself, it is *still* a source of great inspiration, and it is still a beautiful mystery. Our bodies are not what we think they are. When examined closely with the tool of samādhi, they possibly have only the qualities of sat, cit, and ānanda.

So whenever we practice yoga we take another look. We look again for the first time at our breath, and we feel it flow through the nostrils. We examine our thumbs, our fingers and hands, our arms, feet, and our legs. We feel the mouth, and we sense that skin is all over the body. We look once again at each other, at the world, and at the mind—all anew and fresh, without the preconceptions that come from past experience. Looking into the mirror of yoga we see there is something deep, completely mysterious, extraordinarily joyous, and most of all very familiar.

Acknowledgments

THIS BOOK IS the result of the kindness and endless patience of the wonderful people who surround and inspire me. The foremost of these is my beloved wife and muse, Mary Taylor, who sees the best in me and who has worked tirelessly in organizing and editing the text. It was she who lit the fire, which led to the creation of the original *Yoga Matrix* audiotapes from which this book was derived. Thanks are due to Tami Simon and the people of Sounds True who drew *Yoga Matrix* out of me. Thank you also Sara Bercholz of Shambhala Publications, who has had unwavering enthusiasm for my work, and for others at Shambhala who have helped in the editing and production of this book. Elizabeth Gregg, who types like lightning, did the original transcription from the CDs. My endless gratitude goes to Gabe Freeman for not being reducible to or reducing himself to any theory.

Shri K. Pattabhi Jois of Mysore, my primary guru, tied together all of the yogas into one for me. Shri B. K. S. Iyengar allowed me to feel and embody transmuted emotion. Matsuoka Roshi of Chicago was my early inspiration and grounding in the unbearable simplicity of yoga as Zen practice. A. C. Bhaktivedanta Swami taught me the ins and outs of the paradoxes of religious thought. My mind is always renewed and inspired by the work of Chögyam Trungpa Rinpoche and the brilliant light and depth of Buddhist teachings.

Special thanks are due to Susan Chiocchi for the brilliant illustrations, which are drawings of the undrawable.

And finally I would like to acknowledge all the students and teachers of the Yoga Workshop in Boulder, Colorado, who have listened with such attention for all these years.

Sanskrit Pronunciation Guide

Sanskrit is the language in which the hymns of ancient India, the Vedas, and the many thousands of subsequent texts and epics were composed. Though it is no longer considered a spoken language, it is still used extensively in many of the yoga traditions of Asia as a sacred language for chanting, mantra, and the study of philosophy. The word *Sanskrit* means "constructed," "polished," or "perfected." The pronunciation, grammar, and rules for linking its words were crafted and tuned to create and maintain a basic, underlying humming resonant quality, which proves to be entrancing and joyous to the practiced chanter. It requires a precise articulation of the tongue and use of breath as well as tone in order to create the sounds well. These pronunciation guidelines will give a close approximation to the correct sound. The simple vowels (*a, i, u*) may be either short (one beat as *a* without a mark above) or long (two beats with a horizontal line above, as in *ā*). The diphthongs (*e, ai, o, au*) are also long (two beats). Consonants each have five different forms of pronunciation depending on the positioning of the tongue making them: guttural, palatal, cerebral, dental, or labial. These sounds do not all directly correspond to sounds within the English language or to the alphabet, so the Roman transliteration has diacritical markings to indicate which Sanskrit sound the letter indicates.

Vowels

a - pronounced like "a" in pizza

i - pronounced like "ee" in squeeze

u - pronounced like "oo" in smooth

ā, ī, ū - pronounced as above, but held for two beats

ai - pronounced like "a" in say (natural diphthong, two beats)

e - pronounced like "e" in they (natural diphthong, two beats)

o - pronounced like "o" in open (natural diphthong, two beats)

au - pronounced like "ow" in how (natural diphthong, two beats)

Consonants

The consonants are grouped by the sounds made due to the position and placement of the tongue in the mouth. There are five positions with five sounds at each position. The second and fourth sound in each position are aspirated. The fifth sound is the nasal "mm" sound with the tongue remaining in the correct position for the group.

Gutturals: ka, kha, ga, gha, nā
The sound is back in the throat and the tongue does not touch the palate.

Palatals: ca, cha, ja, jha, ña
The sound is pushed up into the palate and the tongue lightly touches the mid-hard palate.

Cerebrals: ṭa, ṭha, ḍa, ḍha, ṇa
The sound stays back in the sinuses and the tip of the tongue is pulled down after touching the center point of the palate.

Dentals; ta, tha, da, dha, na
The sound is forward in the mouth and the tongue touches the back of the upper front teeth.

Labials: pa, pha, ba, bha, ma
The sound is forward in the mouth and is produced by the opening of the lips. The tongue is neutral.

Common transliteration markings are:

h after a consonant - the aspirant sound that appears in English between certain palatal and guttural sounds such as "top hat" (aspirant *p*) and cab house (aspirant *b*).

c - pronounced like "ch" in churn

ṛ - pronounced like "r" in brook

s - pronounced like "s" in synthesis

ś - pronounced like "sh" in shock

ṣ - pronounced like "sh" in sheer

ṅ - pronounced like "n" in bunion

ṁ - pronounced like "n" in uncle

jñ - pronounced like "ghee-yah"

h - pronounced like "ha"

ḥ - pronounced with a soft echo of the preceding vowel

Chanting

Chanting is an integral part of the yoga tradition; reflecting on the meaning of the words of the chant while the sound resonates through the body can have a transformative effect. Traditional orthodox chants are Vedic (meaning that their source is the early period of the Vedas), in which case there are very precise and specific conventions that must be followed when chanting. In addition to applying the general rules of Sanskrit pronunciation (vowel length, placement of tongue, and so on), Vedic chanting has only three tones allowed: the middle tone, the half-step up, and a full-step down. This variation in tone is called the *svara* and it is predetermined within the text. With other forms of classical chanting there is room for creativity—not in terms of pronunciation, but in terms of the tune. An audio recording of the seven chants below, some of which are Vedic and others which are not, is available for download at www. shambhala.com/MirrorofYoga.

Ganesha Mantra

g̱aṇānāṁ̎ tvā g̱aṇapa̍tigaṁ havāmahe

ḵaviṁ ka̍vī̱nāmu̍pamaśra̍vastamam |

jy̱eṣṯarājaṁ̱ brahma̍ṇāṁ brahmaṇaspata̱ ā na̍ḥ

śṛ̱ṇvannū̱tibhi̍ssīda̱ sāda̍nam ||

Oṁ

We invoke thee, O leader of all the hosts. The wisest of the wise. The Sage of Sages with treasures beyond measure. The King of Brilliance. The lead chanter of prayers. Come with your blessings, listen to our prayers. Have a seat in our sacred space.

Invocation to the Guru and Patañjali

vande gurūṇāṁ caraṇāravinde
sandarśita svātma sukhāva bodhe
niḥśreyase jāṅgalikāyamāne
saṁsāra hālāhala moha śantyai
Oṁ

I bow to the two lotus feet of the (plurality of) Gurus,
which awaken insight
Into the happiness of pure Being, which are the complete
absorption into joy,
The jungle physician, eliminating the delusion
Caused by the poison of Saṁsāra (conditioned existence).

ābāhu puruṣākāraṁ
śaṅkha cakrāsi dhāriṇam |
sahasra śirsaṁ śvetaṁ
praṇamāmi patañjalim ||
Oṁ

I prostrate before the sage Patañjali who has thousands of radiant,
White heads (as the divine serpent, Ananta) and who has, as far
As his arms, assumed a human form, holding a conch shell
(divine sound),
A wheel (a discus of light or time), and a sword (discrimination).

Meditation on the Serpent of Infinity

maṇi bhrātphaṇā sahasravighṛtaviśvaṁ
bharāmaṇḍalāyānantāya nāgarājāya namaḥ

Salutations to the king of the Nagas,
To the infinite, to the bearer of the maṇḍala,
Who spreads out the universe with thousands
Of hooded heads, set with blazing, effulgent jewels.

Two Verses from the Gītā Dhyānam

vasudeva sutaṁ devaṁ kaṁsa cāṇūra mardanaṁ ǀ
devakī paramānandaṁ kṛṣnaṁ vande jagadgurum ǀǀ 5

I adore Kṛṣṇa, the god who is the Son of Vasudeva, the destroyer of Kamsa and Canura,
The supreme joy of Devaki and the Guru of the whole creation.

mūkaṁ karoti vācālaṁ paṅguṁ laṅghayate girim ǀ
yatkṛpā tamhaṁ vande paramānanda mādhavaṁ ǀǀ 8

I *salute Madhava, the supreme joy, by whose grace the dumb speak eloquently and the lame cross mountains.*

Verse from the Bhagavad Gītā on Fire

brahmārpaṇaṁ brahma havir
brahmāgnau brahmaṇā hutam ǀ
brahmaiva tena gantavyaṁ
brahmakarmasamādhinā
Oṁ

Brahman is the offering, Brahman is the oblation, poured out by Brahman into the fire of Brahman, Brahman is to be attained by one who contemplates the action of Brahman.

Heart of the Gītā

ahaṁ sarvasya prabhavo
mattaḥ sarvaṁ pravartate
iti matvā bhajante māṁ
budhā bhāvasamanvitāḥ

I am the origin of all.
All proceeds from Me.
Thinking in this way, those who are wide awake
Worship me with concentrated meditation

maccittā madgataprāṇā
bodhayantaḥ parasparam
kathayantaśca māṁ nityaṁ
tuṣyanti ca ramanti ca

Those who think of Me, who absorb their lives in Me,
Enlightening each other
And speaking of Me constantly,
They are content and they rejoice.

teṣāṁ satatayuktānā,
bhajatāṁ prītipūrvakam
dadāmi buddhiyogaṁ taṁ
yena mām upayānti te

To those who are always linking in Yoga,
Those who worship Me with love,

I give the yoga of discrimination
By which they come to Me.

teṣāṁ evānukampārtham
aham ajñānajaṁ tamaḥ
nāśayāmy ātmabhāvastho
jñānadīpena bhāsvatā

Out of compassion for them,
I, who dwell within their own hearts,
Destroy the darkness born of ignorance
With the shining lamp of knowledge.

Closing Chant

svasti prajābhyaḥ paripālayantām
nyāyena mārgeṇa mahīṁ mahīśāḥ |
gobrāhmaṇebhyaḥ śubhamastu nityaṁ
lokāsamastā sukhino bhavantu ||
kāle varṣatu parjanyaḥ pṛthivī sasyaśālinī |
deśoyaṁ kṣobharahito brāhmaṇā santu nirbhayāḥ ||

May all of humankind be happy and well.
May the great noble lords protect the earth in every way by the path of just virtue.
May there be perpetual joy for those who know the real nature of things.
May all the worlds be happy.
May the rains fall on time, and may the earth yield its produce in abundance.
May this country be free from disturbances, and may the knowers of the truth be free from fear.

ākāśa. sky

apas. water. river

earth. muladaka. prthivi

GLOSSARY

ahaṁkāra. The ego function, the I-maker.

ahiṁsā. Nonharming or nonviolence. The first of the yamas.

ākāśa. Sky, space, or nonobstructive openness.

anāhata cakra. "The wheel of unstruck (sound)" or the heart cakra.

ānanda. Joy, bliss, the intrinsic nature of pure awareness.

anusvāra. The dot that is placed above letters within Sanskrit writing (Devanagari) to indicate the dissolution of a nasal "mmm" sound into a place just above the soft palate.

apāna. The pattern of the inner life breath that governs exhaling. The physical and neurological patterns within the body associated with dropping, grounding, relaxing, stabilizing, and eliminating waste.

apas. Water, river.

āsana. Arrangement and alignment of the body so that meditation can occur. the third limb of the eightfold yoga system.

aṣṭāṅga. Eight limbs; used in reference to the eight-limbed path of yoga that leads to discriminating awareness and liberation. Aṣṭāṅga Vinyasa yoga is also a popular form of yoga āsana practice that involves a flowing, meditative form of āsana practice in which postures and movement are linked together with breathing, bandhas, mudrā, and gaze.

ātman. The Self; pure consciousness.

avidyā.   Not-knowing or ignorance; the basic cause of suffering because it is the confusion of impermanent process with pure consciousness.

Bhagavad Gītā.   The "Song of God," the story of Arjuna, a warrior, who is taught yoga by his charioteer, Kṛṣṇa,

bhakti.   Devotion, the practice of devotion. Bhakti is a school of yoga that emphasizes surrender to, contemplation of, and service to God as the supreme Beloved.

bindu.   Droplet, point, or seed.

Brahman.   The whole, the true nature of all things, the ground of Being; pure consciousness, joy, and truth; in the Vedānta it is the absolute truth.

buddhi.   Intelligence, the principle of mind that reveals context and connections, the context maker. *Vikalpa   Sankalpa thinking — aspiration — imagine — compost*

cakra.   Wheel or energy center along the central axis, a point where *Manas mind* the mind can easily enter into contemplation of the strong flow of sensation associated with the particular quality of the cakra.

central axis of the body.   The midline, the plumb line through the body; corresponding to the subtle suṣumnā nāḍī and considered to be the main channel or nāḍī of the subtle body.

cit-acit granthi.   The knot of the unconscious and pure consciousness; another term for the ego process.

citta.   The entire mind in its most inclusive sense.

devatā.   A goddess or a god.

dharma.   Duty, obligation, religion, the fundamental quality of a thing, one's calling in life, the glue that holds things together, the constituent factors that come together to form a particular experience.

dhyāna.   Meditation, the level of contemplation when the attention flows smoothly as its object, when conflict with the background of the object has ceased.

duḥkha.   Suffering, frustration; literally a "bad hole" in a wheel, which *BAD HOLE* would give a bumpy ride.

sankalpa - unified constructions
vikalpa - divided constructions

Gaṇeśa. The elephant-headed god of Indian mythology associated with keen intelligence and the removal of obstacles. He is the embodiment of much of the esoteric and secret teachings of haṭha and tantric yoga. He holds the key to the ever-elusive mūlabandha.

guṇas. Energetic strands of creative energy that are woven together in varying proportion to form the underlying structure of all things. Each thread has a distinctive characteristic. Tamas (tamasic) is fixed, slow, sluggish, thick—the thesis. Rajas (rajasic) is fiery, strong, fast, and active—the antithesis. Sattva is stable, smooth, integrated, balanced, and sweet—synthesis.

haṭha yoga. A general term for forms of yoga that include physical practices. *Ha* means "sun" and *ṭha* means "moon"; haṭha yoga is the joining together and interpenetration of opposite patterns. Esoterically haṭha is a forcing together of prāṇa and apāna to awaken the kuṇḍalinī.

Haṭha Yoga Pradīpikā. A primary yoga text from between the fourteenth and sixteenth centuries C.E., which describes the technical practices of kuṇḍalinī awakening and absorption of the mind in samādhi.

iḍā. The moon channel (nāḍī) or nostril, which is associated with a pluralistic, feminine, cooling breath within the body.

indriyas. The senses.

Jeweled Net of Indra. The net of illusion said to be cast over people by the god Indra; a net that causes the confusion of what is real, lasting (pure consciousness, or puruṣa) with what is unreal, impermanent (creative energy and forms, or prakṛti). One can be free of the net by looking very closely at it.

jñāna. Knowledge; ultimately knowledge of reality.

karma yoga. The yoga of work.

kuṇḍalinī. The great supporting serpent said to lie coiled and dormant just above the center of the pelvic floor. In her dormant state she blocks the entrance into the suṣumnā nāḍī, keeping the internal breath out of the liberating middle path.

Mahābharata. The great epic story of Indian mythology that includes, as part of it, the Bhagavad Gītā.

mahāśakti. The great śakti or creative energy.

manas. The mind as the organizer of perception, producing unified constructions (saṅkalpa) and divided constructions (vikalpa).

maṇḍala. A circular geometric pattern used as a sacred space or temple for meditation, or to collect together the particular qualities of a deity.

mantra. A phrase or sound, which is chanted in repetition and used for collecting the attention for concentration or meditation and to clarify and focus the mind.

mudrā. A sealing or pressing together to make self-contained form a form or flow of a pattern for meditation. Mudrās can be formed with the fingers or with the body as gestures and expressions of deep internal states. Internal mudrās are used to open the central channel.

mūlādhāra cakra. The cakra or energy center associated with the pelvic floor. It is the "holder of the root" and is associated with the element earth.

niyamas. The internal practices and observances. Five are mentioned in the *Yoga Sūtra*.

Patañjali. The composer of the *Yoga Sūtra*. Patañjali is said to be half divine serpent, Ādi Śeṣa, and half human; the lower part of his body is represented as a coiled snake, the upper part as a four-armed human, with a cobra's body rising up along his back and forming a hood of an endless number of radiant heads.

piṅgalā. The solar channel (nāḍī), beginning in the right nostril and associated with the clear, singular focus and heat within the body.

prakṛti. The universal creative energy that forms any object of awareness no matter how subtle. Prakṛti is not conscious, and its products are always impermanent.

prāṇa. The vital or internal breath that organizes all perceptions and influences the moments of the mind. It has many internal functions.

The most obvious are inhaling controlled by the prāṇa (a subcategory by the same name) and exhaling controlled by the apāna.

prāṇāyāma. Meditative breathing practices that gradually decondition the breathing habits and patterns associated with a distracted mind. The practices stretch or extend the inhale, the exhale, and the suspensions between them, allowing the sensations and emotions associated with each phase of the breath to become objects of meditation.

pratyāhāra. The nongrasping of objects by the senses in which the mind ceases to form the appearance of separate, continuous objects within the fields of the senses. This is the fifth limb of the eightfold yoga system.

pṛthivī. Earth, externally that which we all share and stand upon, and internally the quality of stability, fixedness, and complete cohesion.

puruṣa. Pure consciousness; the actual true being for whom creative energy exists within the Sāṁkhya system.

rajas (rajasic). The component of creative energy that is fiery, strong, fast, and active and which forms an antithesis to the dull and the fixed.

Rāmāyaṇa. The great epic that tells the story of Rama.

rasa. Juice, essence, flavor, proportion.

ṛṣis. The seers who sang the descriptive and lyrical poetry that became the hymns of the Vedas.

sahasrāra. The thousand-petaled lotus flower said to be accessed at the crown of the head. It is not considered to be a cakra; rather it stands above as the vast universal array of awakened beings and realms. At its base, just above the root of the palate, is a receptacle in the form of the moon or an ocean, which collects nectar.

Sāṁkhya. Probably the first major, complete system of philosophical thought appearing in the post-Vedic period, during the time of the composition of the early Upaniṣads. First taught by the sage Kapila, it posits the idea that puruṣa (pure consciousness) and the prakṛti (creative energy or all that manifests—thoughts, feelings, sensations, objects, sentient beings, ideas, and so on) are separate, yet prakṛti exists to bind and then to reveal puruṣa.

Sāṁkhya Kārikā. The primary and most detailed text of the Saṁkhya philosophy; written by Īśvara Kṛṣṇa.

saṁsāra. Conditioned existence, represented as a wheel of suffering turned by the relentless flow of ignorant habits, karma, and reactions.

saṁskāra. Habitual patterns within the body and mind (and consequently in action). These are formed when deep sensation patterns within prāṇa become superimposed with memories and concepts.

saṅkalpa. To think or to imagine into composite wholes, intentions, desires, and aspirations.

Sanskṛt. The sacred, constructed, and polished language in which most ancient yogic and Indian philosophy texts are written. Though it is still used within the Hindu and yogic traditions when studying texts and chanting, it is not generally used as a spoken language.

sattva (sattvic). Beingness, or stable, smooth, balanced, bright, integrated.

sudhā. Nectar of immortality.

sukha. Happiness, ease; derived from the concept of a good hole in a wheel.

suṣumnā nāḍī. The central channel of the body, the esoteric middle path which is visualized as a bright hollow reed or tube. When opened so that the prāṇa flows in it, it consumes time and space.

tamas (tamasic). Slow, sluggish, thick, dull, fixed as in a thesis.

tantra (tantric). A large group of practices and schools that have existed in and around the orthodox Vedic schools of practice.

tapas. Heat; the heat caused from work.

Upaniṣads. Primary philosophy texts that followed the Vedas. There are 10 principle Upaniṣads considered essential to the study of yoga. They define the early period of the Vedānta, or the end of the Vedic period in Indian philosophy. Later Upaniṣads, composed over a period of twenty-five hundred years, bring the total number of them to more than 108.

vairāgyam. Dispassion, letting go, letting be, release.

vāyu. Wind, often referring to the different forms of prāṇa inside the body.

Vedānta. The various forms of non-dual philosophy concerned with direct experience of truth and liberation from conditioned existence. Vedānta arose in the period of philosophical exploration that followed the Vedas.

Vedas (Vedic). Ancient hymns memorized and chanted to this day by priests. They form the basis for rituals, sacrifices, philosophies, and cultural patterns that today fall under the broad term *Hindu*.

vikalpa. To split into categories; the function of the mind that imagines all sorts of constructions.

viveka khyātiḥ. Discriminating awareness. The ability to discriminate between that which is real, permanent, and considered to be pure consciousness, and that which is unreal, impermanent, and considered to be creative energy.

yamas. Ethical standards of a balanced yoga practice; delineated in a number of yogic texts, including the *Yoga Sūtra*.

Yoga Sūtra. A primary yoga text that is a collection of aphorisms organized into four books (pādas) and that describes the process of yoga. It is said to have been composed by the sage Patañjali.

INDEX

prana - internal breath

About the Author

Richard Freeman began the study of yoga in 1968 at the Chicago Zen Center while earning an MA in philosophy. Over the course of the next ten years he traveled extensively and lived in Asia, studying Indian and Buddhist philosophy, Sufism, yoga āsana, prāṇāyāma, and meditation. His early years with āsana practice were deeply influenced by B. K. S Iyengar. Later Freeman found an integrative vision of the practice in the Aṣṭāṅga Vinyasa yoga tradition as taught to him by his primary teacher K. Pattabhi Jois. He currently travels throughout the world teaching yoga, philosophy, and meditation. He has produced three best-selling āsana practice DVDs and several highly acclaimed CDs on the subjects of chanting, prāṇāyāma, and basic yoga philosophy, including *The Yoga Matrix,* a CD set that served as the springboard for this book. Freeman is also the founder and owner of the Yoga Workshop in Boulder, Colorado, where he teaches and lives with his family. For more information about Richard's teaching, online recordings, and other work, you can find him at www.yogaworkshop.com.

About the Illustrator

Susan Chiocchi, BFA, worked as a professional illustrator for many years and now has a private healing practice in Boulder, Colorado, where she lives with her family. She has studied and practiced yoga for more than twenty years, has been a student of Richard's since 1986, and teaches at the Yoga Workshop. Susan is a certified Reiki master teacher, has a diploma in Brennan Healing Science, and continues her studies of the human energy body in relation to healing, yoga, and consciousness through yoga and Bön Buddhist studies.